Left Main Coronary Artery Disease

D1322187

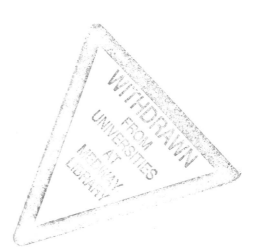

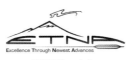

Ferrarotto Hospital   *ETNA Foundation*   *University of Catania*   Società Italiana
di Cardiologia Invasiva

Corrado Tamburino

Left Main Coronary Artery Disease

A Practical Guide for the Interventional Cardiologist

In collaboration with
Maria Elena Di Salvo
Alessio La Manna
Davide Capodanno

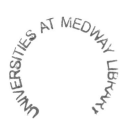

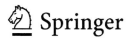 Springer

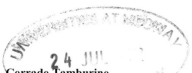

Corrado Tamburino
Full Professor of Cardiology, Director of Postgraduate School of Cardiology,
Chief Cardiovascular Department and Director Cardiology Division,
Ferrarotto Hospital, University of Catania, Catania, Italy

In collaboration with
Maria Elena Di Salvo, Alessio La Manna
Co-Directors Interventional Cardiology, Cardiology Division, Ferrarotto Hospital, Catania,
Italy, and
Davide Capodanno
Research Fellow, Chair of Cardiology, University of Catania, Catania, Italy

The authors gratefully acknowledge the valuable technical and scientific support in the realization of this volume offered by:
Alfredo R. Galassi, Salvatore Davide Tomasello, Francesco Tagliareni, Piera Capranzano, Dario Seminara, Anna Caggegi, Giombattista Barrano, Marco Miano, Glauco Cincotta, Laura Basile and Associazione Cuore e Ricerca

ISBN 978-88-470-1429-9   e-ISBN 978-88-470-1430-5

DOI 10.1007/978-88-4701430-5

Springer Dordrecht Heidelberg London Milan New York

Library of Congress Control Number: 2009927094

Drawings by: Giombattista Barrano

Typesetting: Compostudio, Cernusco s/N (Milan), Italy
Printing and binding: Arti Grafiche Nidasio, Assago (Milan), Italy
Printed in Italy

Springer-Verlag Italia S.r.l, Via Decembrio 28, I-20137 Milan, Italy
Springer is part of Springer Science+Business Media (www.springer.com)

This volume is dedicated to Dr. Ambrogio Mazzeo,
general manager of my hospital,
for his merits and empathy towards
patients with heart disease.

Corrado Tamburino

Preface

When I decided to rise to the challenge of writing a manual on the percutaneous treatment of the left main coronary artery (LMCA), I tried to stand in the shoes of my readers, namely interventional cardiologists who wish to treat these types of lesion, but who refrain from doing so owing to a lack of confidence due to technical and procedural reasons.

LMCA angioplasty is often perceived as an extremely complex procedure with a high incidence of periprocedural complications, which should always be avoided in the presence of the evidence suggested by guidelines; this, in turn, leaves the surgeon to address the brunt of the issues related to treatment.

In actual fact, though, the application of percutaneous coronary intervention (PCI) to select cases has proven to be safe and effective. This is corroborated by the latest evidence in the literature and it is quite likely that the proportion of LMCA lesions treated with PCI (which currently accounts for about one-third of cases in Europe) is bound to rise in the near future.

Regardless of whether the indications are appropriate, which is currently being debated and encouraging the design of new randomized trials, in most cases the strictly procedural issues can be overcome by a skilled interventional cardiologist with the aid of suitable materials and techniques.

The objective of this manual is to provide quick reference and a highly practical and useful approach for cardiologists who wish to gain greater insight into this particular field of coronary interventional cardiology and to learn how to identify the diverse presentations of the disease, choose the most appropriate interventional strategies, and apply these swiftly and with ease.

Catania, April 2008   **Corrado Tamburino**

Acknowledgements

The authors thank Martina Patanè and Claudia Tamburino, students of the course of medicine, University of Catania, Italy, for their valuable support.

Contents

3   Morpho-functional Assessment of Left Main Coronary Artery Disease

4   Left Main Coronary Artery Percutaneous Interventions: Materials and Techniques

List of Authors and Contributors

Corrado Tamburino
Full Professor of Cardiology
Director of Postgraduate School
of Cardiology
Chief Cardiovascular Department
Director Cardiology Division
Ferrarotto Hospital
University of Catania
Catania, Italy

Maria Elena Di Salvo
Co-Director Interventional
Cardiology
Cardiology Division
Ferrarotto Hospital
Catania, Italy

Alessio La Manna
Co-Director Interventional
Cardiology
Cardiology Division
Ferrarotto Hospital
Catania, Italy

Davide Capodanno
Research Fellow
Chair of Cardiology
University of Catania
Catania, Italy

Piera Capranzano
Postgraduate School of Cardiology
University of Catania
Catania, Italy

Alfredo R. Galassi
Associate Professor of Cardiology
Postgraduate School of Cardiology
University of Catania
Co-Director Interventional
Cardiology
Cardiology Division
Ferrarotto Hospital
Catania, Italy

Salvatore Davide Tomasello
Postgraduate School of Cardiology
University of Catania
Catania, Italy

Francesco Tagliareni
Postgraduate School of Cardiology
University of Catania
Catania, Italy

Dario Seminara
Postgraduate School of Cardiology
University of Catania
Catania, Italy

Anna Caggegi
Postgraduate School of Cardiology
University of Catania
Catania, Italy

Giombattista Barrano
Postgraduate School of Cardiology
University of Catania
Catania, Italy

Marco Miano
Postgraduate School of Cardiology
University of Catania
Catania, Italy

Glauco Cincotta
Postgraduate School of Cardiology
University of Catania
Catania, Italy

Laura Basile
Executive PA
Chair of Cardiology
University of Catania
ETNA Foundation
Catania, Italy

Abbreviations

ACS	acute coronary syndrome
ARC	Academic Research Consortium
BMS	bare metal stents
CABG	coronary artery bypass grafting
CAD	coronary artery disease
CASS	Coronary Artery Surgery Study
CCTA	coronary computed tomographic angiography
CI	confidence interval
CMR	cardiovascular magnetic resonance
CMRA	coronary magnetic resonance angiography
CT	computerized tomography
2D	two-dimensional
3D	three-dimensional
DELFT	Drug-Eluting stent for LeFT Main (registry)
DES	drug-eluting stents
DMV	distal main vessel
FFR	fractional flow reserve
HR	hazard ratio
IABP	intra-aortic balloon pump
ICPS	Institut Cardiovasculaire Paris-Sud
ISR	in-stent restenosis
IVUS	intravascular ultrasound
LAD	left anterior descending artery
LCX	left circumflex artery
LE MANS	Unprotected Left Main Stenting Versus Bypass Surgery (study)
LMCA	left main coronary artery
LVEF	left ventricular ejection fraction
MACCE	major adverse cerebro-cardiovascular event

MACE	major adverse cardiac events
MB	main branch
MLA	minimum lumen area
MLD	minimum lumen diameter
MSA	minimum stent area
MSCT	multi-slice computed tomography
MV	main vessel
NSTEMI	non-ST-segment elevation myocardial infarction
OFDI	optical frequency domain imaging
OCT	optical coherence tomography
OR	odds ratio
PAR-1	thrombin protease-activated receptor
PCI	percutaneous coronary intervention
PES	paclitaxel-eluting stent
PET	positron emission tomography
PMV	proximal main vessel
QCA	quantitative coronary analysis
RCA	right coronary artery
RESEARCH	Rapamycin-Eluting Stent Evaluated At Rotterdam Cardiology Hospital
RI	ramus intermedius
RR	relative risk
RVD	reference vessel diameter
SB	side branch
SES	sirolimus-eluting stents
SICI-GISE	Società Italiana di Cardiologia Invasiva - Gruppo Italiano Studi Emodinamici
SKS	simultaneous kissing stents
ST	stent thrombosis
SYNTAX	Synergy between PCI with Taxus and Cardiac Surgery (trial)
TEE	transesophageal echocardiography
TLR	target lesion revascularization
T-SEARCH	Taxus-Stent Evaluated At Rotterdam Cardiology Hospital
TVR	target vessel revascularization
ULMCA	unprotected left main coronary artery
ULTIMA	Unprotected Left Main Trunk Intervention Multicenter Assessment

Anatomy

1.1
Normal Anatomy

The left main coronary artery (LMCA) normally arises from the aorta, above the left cusp of the aortic valve and just below the sino-tubular ridge. As it exits from the aortic sinus, it enters the leftward margin of the transverse sinus, being positioned between the left atrial appendage and the pulmonary trunk. It typically runs for 1 to 25 mm and then bifurcates into the left anterior descending artery (LAD) and the left circumflex artery (LCX). Its branches usually supply a larger volume of myocardium, including most of the left ventricle, the muscular ventricular septum, and the supero-lateral papillary muscle of the mitral valve, as well as giving branches to the left atrium, and in just under half the population also supplying the artery of the sinus node. In around one-quarter of the population, the LMCA also gives rise to an inter-mediate branch, and in rare cases to two intermediate arteries.

Interventional cardiologists are well aware of the fact that there are different anatomical LMCA phenotypes that generally fall into this general scheme. However, these phenotypes are capable of having a major impact in determining the approach to percutaneous treatment of coronary atherosclerotic disease.

While surgery is not dependent on choices linked to LMCA anatomy, the interventional strategy and materials may vary depending on LMCA anatomy, its interaction with the ascending aorta, the gauge, the length, and bifurcation architecture.

To date no attempt has yet been made to systematically classify LMCA anatomy. The literature offers scarce specific information and there are no studies on how frequently the various anatomical conformations occur in the patient population referred to catheterization labs. In the light of the practical objectives set in this manual, an effort has been made to fill this gap through a systematic approach using a series of definitions based on practice and experience.

There are five variables defining the LMCA from a strictly morphological viewpoint, namely, the angle of take-off from the aorta, course, designation of bifurcation, length, and diameter. The most useful angiographic views when studying either a normal or pathological LMCA anatomy are the anteroposterior, caudal anteroposterior, left anterior oblique with cranial tilt, and cranial left anterior oblique.

1.1.1
Angle of Take-off

The LMCA angle of take-off is the angle between the aortic lumen and the coronary ostial lumen. It may be acute (Fig. 1.1a, b), right (Fig. 1.2a, b), or obtuse (Fig. 1.3a, b).

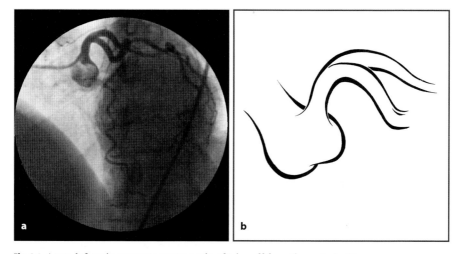

Fig. 1.1 Acute left main coronary artery angle of take-off from the aorta (**a, b**)

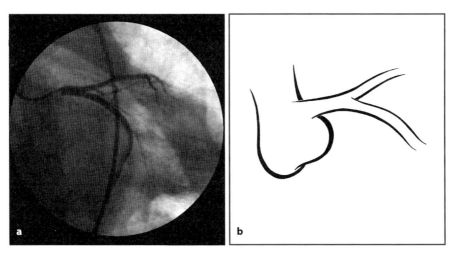

Fig 1.2 Right left main coronary artery angle of take-off from the aorta (**a**, **b**)

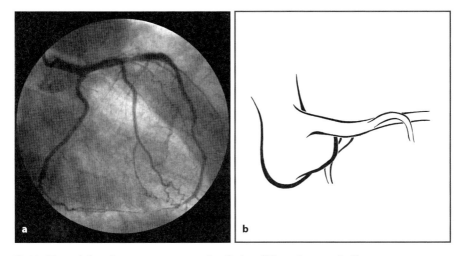

Fig 1.3 Obtuse left main coronary artery angle of take-off from the aorta (**a**, **b**)

1.1.2
Course

The course of the LMCA may be dichotomized as *angulated* or *straight* according to the presence or absence of any angle located either in the proximal, middle, or distal segment of the coronary segment (Fig. 1.4a, b).

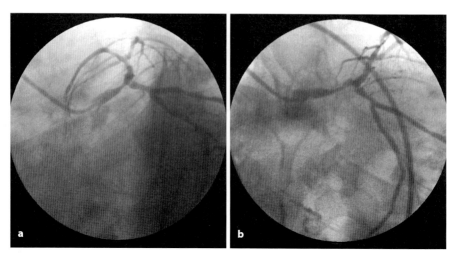

Fig. 1.4 a Straight course of the left main coronary artery. **b** Distal angulation (prebifurcational) of the left main coronary artery

1.1.3
Designation of Bifurcation (Fig. 1.5)

In the absence of three-dimensional image reconstruction for all angiograms, the best way to achieve reliable measurement of the angles between the various segments is to perform it in the angiographic view, in which the foreshortening of the three segments is minimal. As previously suggested [1], the angle

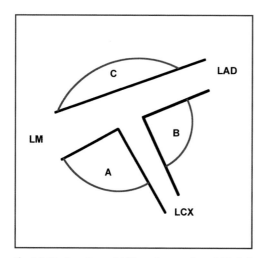

Fig. 1.5 Designation of bifurcation angles; *LM*, left main coronary artery; *LAD*, left anterior descending artery; *LCX*, left circumflex artery

between the distal LMCA and LCX proximal trunk is called angle A. This angle is deemed to have an influence on the accessibility of the side branch. For practical purposes, it may be claimed as acute (Fig. 1.6a, b), right (Fig. 1.7a, b), or obtuse (Fig. 1.8a, b).

Angle B is between the LAD and LCX and has been shown to be related to the impact of side branch occlusion during main branch stenting. Similar to angle A, it may be claimed as acute (Fig. 1.8b), right (Fig. 1.7b), or obtuse

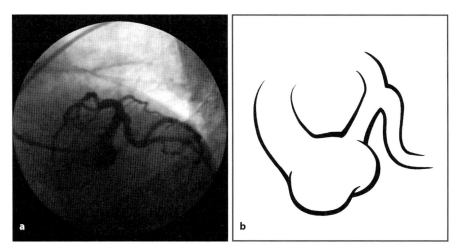

Fig. 1.6 Acute angle of take-off of the left circumflex artery (angle A) (**a, b**)

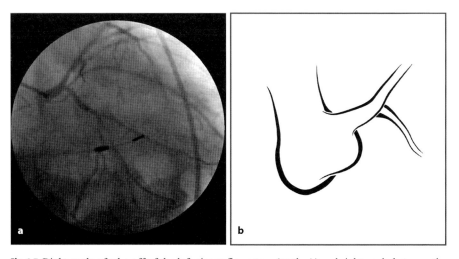

Fig. 1.7 Right angle of take-off of the left circumflex artery (angle A) and right angle between the left anterior descending and left circumflex arteries (angle B) (**a, b**)

(Fig. 1.9). Defining these two angles is essential in order to depict the bifurcation architecture.

Angle C is additionally defined as the angle between the proximal and distal main branch (distal LMCA and LAD, respectively), and for practical purposes it may be treated as a binary variable [absent (Fig. 1.9) or present (Fig. 1.10)].

In our context, it was decided that the best practical method to adopt for the classification of LMCA bifurcation geometry was to develop a theoretical

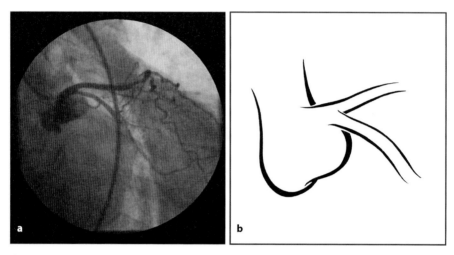

Fig. 1.8 Obtuse angle of take-off of the left circumflex artery (angle A) and acute angle between the left anterior descending and left circumflex (angle B) arteries (**a, b**)

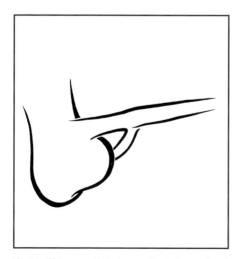

Fig. 1.9 Obtuse angle between the left anterior descending and left circumflex (angle B) arteries; absence of angle between the distal left main coronary artery and the left anterior descending artery (angle C)

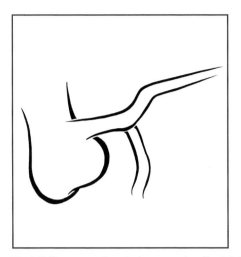

Fig. 1.10 Presence of angle between the distal left main coronary artery and the left anterior descending artery (angle C)

model in which two possibilities are considered. The first one deals with the absence of angle C, in which a type 1 bifurcation is described when angles A and B are acute and obtuse, respectively (Fig. 1.11a); type 2 when angles A and B are both right (Fig. 1.11b), and type 3 when angles A and B are obtuse and acute, respectively (Fig. 1.11c). Conversely, the second one deals with the presence of angle C, in which a type 4 bifurcation is identified when angle A is acute and angle B is obtuse (Fig. 1. 11d), type 5 when angle A is right and angle B is obtuse (Fig. 1.11e), and type 6 when angles A and B are obtuse and right, respectively (Fig. 1.11f).

1.1.4
Length and Diameter

These two parameters are obtained from angiographic quantitative analysis. For convenience, however, a short trunk is considered <8 mm and a long one >15 mm (Fig. 1.12a, b). As for the diameter, an optimal cut-off between large and small is 3.5 mm [2].

Table 1.1 shows the frequency of presentation of these characteristics in a population of 1000 consecutive patients undergoing diagnostic catheterization at our catheterization lab.

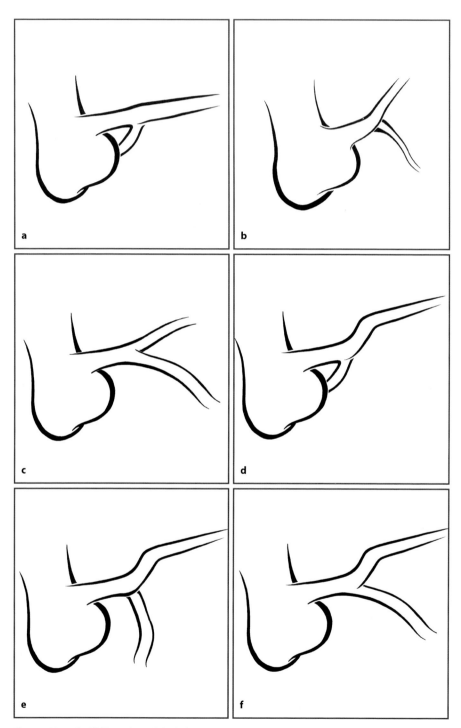

Fig. 1.11 Type 1–6 bifurcation of the left main coronary artery (**a–f**)

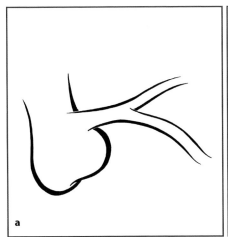 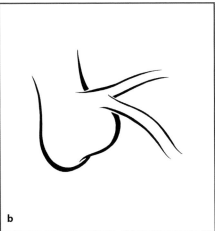

Fig. 1.12 a Long left main coronary artery. **b** Short left main coronary artery

Table 1.1 Presentation of morphological variables defining the left main coronary artery in a patient population of 1000 undergoing diagnostic catheterization

Characteristic	Measurement or frequency of presentation
Length (mm)	11.6 ± 5.0
Diameter (mm)	4.9 ± 1.0
Take-off angle (%)	
Acute	0.8
Straight	67.3
Obtuse	31.9
Course (%)	
Straight	80.4
Proximal angle	8.1
Middle angle	9.8
Distal angle	1.7
Angle A (%)	
Acute	4.5
Straight	36.4
Obtuse	59.1
Angle C (%)	
Absent	88.9
Present	11.1
Bifurcation type (%)	
1	4.0
2	32.2
3	52.6
4	0.6
5	4.1
6	6.5

1.2
Coronary Artery Abnormalities

Coronary artery abnormalities including those of the LMCA have been identified in 1.6% of patients undergoing coronary angiography and in 0.3% of autopsies performed [3]. However, the actual prevalence of this condition in the general population is unknown.

Insight into the congenital abnormalities of the coronary arteries is essential for both cardiologists and cardiothoracic surgeons, owing to the difficulties that may arise during coronary cannulation and to the rare complications that these may cause, as these can lead to a higher cardiovascular risk as a result of the progression of atherosclerosis. They can also lead to diverse symptoms ranging from dyspnea to sudden cardiac death [4].

In 85% of cases these abnormalities are benign and include:
- separate origin of the LAD and LCX from the left sinus of Valsalva
- ectopic origin of the LCX from the right sinus of Valsalva
- ectopic coronary artery originating from the non-coronary sinus
- abnormal origin of a coronary artery from the ascending aorta
- absence of the LCX
- intercoronary shunting.

In turn, the malignant abnormalities can be associated with potentially serious sequelae, such as angina pectoris, acute myocardial infarction, syncope, arrhythmias, congestive heart disease, or sudden death. These abnormalities include:
- abnormal origin of a coronary artery from the pulmonary trunk
- ectopic origin of a coronary artery from the opposite sinus
- single coronary artery
- large coronary fistula.

Abnormalities of the coronary arteries require an accurate diagnosis, proper prognostic stratification and, when necessary, surgical revisions.

For more detailed classification of the LMCA abnormalities, these can be categorized, depending on their origin and course, into [5]:
- abnormal origin from the aorta
- origin from the pulmonary trunk.
    The causes of *abnormal origin from the aorta* are:
- origin of the LMCA from the right sinus of Valsalva; it may take different courses: anterior, posterior, septal, and intra-arterial. The latter, in particular, is associated with the worst prognosis with a high incidence of sudden death
- ectopic origin of the LMCA from the posterior sinus of Valsalva

- origin of the LMCA from the right coronary sinus and junction after several centimeters in the medial third of the anterior descending artery
- LMCA from which only the LAD and a thin hypoplastic LCX originate
- origin of the LMCA from the ascending aorta above the sinus of Valsalva
- origin of the left and right coronary arteries from a single LMCA originating from the right coronary sinus [6].

The *origins of the pulmonary trunk* are divided likewise depending on its course [5]:
- between the aorta and pulmonary trunk
- anterior to the pulmonary trunk
- posterior to the aorta
- posterior to the right ventricular outflow tract within the interventricular septum.

Finally, there is an abnormal presentation of the LMCA where it is totally absent. The LAD and LCX hence originate from separate ostia. In our experience this abnormality occurs in 1.7% of cases.

1.3
Pathological Anatomy of the Left Main Coronary Artery

From a histological viewpoint, the LMCA is a rather peculiar muscular artery. As it originates directly from the aortic wall, it lacks the tunica adventitia at the ostium. In this section the tunica media is extremely rich in smooth muscle cells and elastic tissue and is hence enveloped by the aorta's muscle cells. The elastic component is more abundant here than in any other coronary branch and tends to decrease distally towards the vessel.

1.3.1
Atheromatous Lesions of the Trunk: Distribution and Localization

LMCA stenosis is significant when, by definition, it results in an at least 50% luminal narrowing of the upper vessel. Significant LMCA stenoses occur in 6% of patients undergoing coronary angiography [7]. In some cases familial predisposition has been described [8].

Isolated atheromatous disease of the LMCA is rather unlikely. The vessel's length is an anatomical factor promoting the onset of critical stenoses in the branches originating from it (the shorter the trunk, the greater the exposure to distal coronary atherosclerosis) [9].

Atheromatous lesions of the trunk do not have a homogeneous distribution along the vessel's course. There is an involvement of the distal section in about two-thirds of cases, of the ostial section in about one-quarter of cases, and of the midportion section in the remaining cases [10]. Plaque rupture does not occur with the same frequency in the various sections of the coronary tree, and the critical points are mainly located in the proximal third of the three major coronary branches [11]. Vulnerable plaques are not very frequent in the LMCA or distal coronary portions [12]. This unusual localization may be ascribable to the low shear stress, which the initial portions of the three main coronary vessels are exposed to, owing to the turbulent flow generated by the clash of a high-speed blood flow against the flow dividers at the bifurcation [13].

The necrotic content of the atheromatous plaques is rather low in the trunk and, in particular, in the initial portion, while it reaches a peak at the origin of the LAD and LCX, with a progressive decrease towards the more distal sections. In patients with a long LMCA, the plaque's necrotic core is especially abundant right after the ostium of the two coronary branches originating from it; in patients with a short LMCA, the plaque's necrotic content reaches its maximum about 6 mm after the vessel's origin and then decreases towards the more distal sections of the two branches [13].

1.3.2
Other Pathological Presentations

Large studies on consecutive patients undergoing coronary angiography have shown that the incidence of coronary artery aneurysms varies from 0.3 to 4.9% [14, 15].

LMCA aneurysm is much more uncommon and in a large case history it occurs in only 0.1% of patients undergoing coronary angiography [16].

Coronary artery aneurysm is defined as coronary dilatation that exceeds the diameter of normal adjacent segments or the diameter of the patient's largest coronary vessel by 1.5 times [17]. A more restrictive criterion defines LMCA aneurysm as a dilatation ≥2 times the diameter of the largest coronary vessel or ≥3 times the diameter of a standard catheter (6F) for coronary angiography [18]. LMCA aneurysm is usually associated with multi-vessel atheromatous disease [16], often with severe obstructions adjacent to the aneurysm [19], at times with an involvement of the underlying coronary arteries and bifurcation [20].

Besides atherosclerosis, coronary artery aneurysms can be ascribable to other causes as well. In cases of Kawasaki disease in patients of pediatric age, multiple, widespread, and at times reversible, coronary artery aneurysms are often present; the LMCA can also be more frequently affected in patients with atherosclerotic coronary artery aneurysm [21]. The less frequent causes include traumas, polyarteritis nodosa, systemic lupus erythematosus, Takayasu disease, Marfan syndrome, mycosis, syphilis, and congenital abnormalities. Some forms of aneurysm are due to interventional coronary artery treatment (angioplasty, directional coronary atherectomy) when there is intimal damage and midpoint rupture [22, 23] .

The clinical presentation of coronary artery aneurysm can either be as a sporadic event or as an acute coronary syndrome. Thrombosis resulting from intra-aneurysmal blood stasis due to transformation of the blood flow from laminar to turbulent and the ensuing distal embolization are possible pathogenic mechanisms.

Another cause of severe myocardial ischemia, often leading to sudden death, is dissection of the ascending section of the aorta with a secondary involvement of the coronary artery ostia. In very rare cases the event affects only the LMCA [24, 25].

Without a direct intimal tear, the underlying pathogenic mechanism seems to be rupture of the vasa vasorum in an arterial wall that is rich in peri-adventitial inflammatory infiltrate, with a consequent intramural hematoma in the median tunica and formation of a false lumen, which, as it expands, compresses the real lumen hence causing ischemia. The underlying pathology can either be a vasculitis or abnormal tissue fragility as is the case in Marfan syndrome. At a coronary artery level, cystic medial necrosis is rather uncommon [26].

Finally, the occurrence of a spasm of the LMCA is quite unusual, as it is seldom a spontaneous event and it is usually ascribable to catheter-induced iatrogenic mechanical irritation) [27, 28].

Literature Review

2.1
Data on Surgical Treatment for Unprotected Left Main Coronary Artery Disease

Current guidelines consider surgical treatment as the "gold standard" for unprotected left main coronary artery (ULMCA) revascularization, in the absence of functioning grafts. Indeed, surgery has been widely proven to be more effective in both the short and long term, compared to medical treatment. Starting from the 1960s, many clinical studies comparing surgical versus medical treatment have proved that isolated medical treatment of ULMCA disease is associated with a one-year mortality rate ranging between 24% and 53%. By contrast, surgical treatment significantly reduced mortality, with a 3-year survival rate of 88–93% [29, 30]. Among the surgical series to have provided the rationale for considering surgery the treatment of choice for ULMCA stenosis, the CASS (Coronary Artery Surgery Study) registry is the most extensive prospective study to have performed a comparison between the surgical and medical treatment of left main stenosis, with 1484 patients and a total follow-up of 16 years [31]. This study reported a mean survival of 13.3 years in 1153 patients treated surgically and 6.6 years in the 331 patients treated with medical therapy ($P < 0.0001$). Over the past decade the extensive experience reported in the literature on surgical treatment of the LMCA disease covers more than 11,000 patients, with a hospital mortality of 2.8% and a 1-month mortality ranging from 3% to 4.2% [32–37]. However, of these studies, only two [33, 34] had a follow-up of more than 1 year (2-year mortality: 5–6%) and none had a follow-up of over 2 years. Nevertheless, other surgical experiences have reported less favorable data on mortality and it has been demonstrated that mortality at follow-up is heavily affected by comorbidities. Ellis et al. showed that the 3-year mortality risk varies from 4% in low-risk patients to 40% in high-risk patients with many comorbidities [36]. Although coronary artery bypass grafting (CABG) is associated with high survival among patients with a low surgical risk, it should be noted that this strategy is often associated with high morbidity, due to a considerable incidence of post-operative complications (bleeding, cerebrovascular events, and renal failure are among the most frequently reported).

2.2
Data on Angioplasty and Bare Metal Stents in Unprotected Left Main Coronary Artery

The first cases of percutaneous coronary intervention (PCI) with simple angioplasty of the LMCA were reported by Grüntzig et al. in 1979 [38]. Subsequent experience with simple angioplasty in patients affected by ULMCA disease has given unsatisfactory outcomes, due to a high risk in terms of both mortality and restenosis [39]. It is reasonable to conclude that the poor results of plain angioplasty on main trunk lesions are strongly correlated with the different tissue and structural composition of the LMCA compared to other coronary artery segments: the LMCA ostium is especially rich in elastic fibers, which are probably responsible, following balloon dilation, for an early recoil, which in an acute patient may have catastrophic clinical consequences. The introduction of bare metal stents (BMS) has revamped the role of PCI and increased the use of percutaneous strategies for this particular subgroup of lesions. The use of stents for the treatment of ULMCA has made it possible to partly overcome the limits of plain old balloon angioplasty. Several studies have been carried out to assess the feasibility, efficacy, and safety of left main stenting with BMS. The results reported in these studies are extremely variable, reflecting the great variety of patients included and lesions treated in these different series. Overall, 30-day mortality varies from 0% to 14% and long-term mortality (1–2 years) from 3% to 31% [40–45]. The high mortality reported in some studies is ascribable to the rather high number of patients considered inoperable, or undergoing revascularization in emergency conditions. The ULTIMA (Unprotected Left Main Trunk Intervention Multicenter Assessment) registry, one of the most extensive studies on ULMCA stenting with BMS, reported, in 279 patients, an in-hospital mortality rate of 13.7% and a 1-year mortality of 24.2% [41]. Forty-six per cent of patients were considered inoperable or at high surgical risk, and this is the subgroup with the most cases of death. On the other hand, the subgroup of low-risk patients had no cases of periprocedural death, and overall 1-year mortality was reasonably low (3.4%) [41]. Other studies have reported consistent data showing excellent results, both immediately and in the long term, in patients either considered to be ideal candidates for surgery or electively treated. The Korean experience, one of the largest series of PCI with

BMS in ULMCA, has reported a long-term mortality of 7.4% in a population of 270 patients with preserved ventricular function [44]. Despite the high success rate in terms of mortality associated with the use of BMS, in patients also eligible for CABG, all the series of PCI with BMS in ULMCA report a high incidence of re-intervention, ranging between 15% and 34% (at 1–2 years' follow-up). Overall mortality and the high percentage of re-intervention reported in these studies affected the guidelines released in 2001 and 2005. Indeed, European and US guidelines indicate ULMCA PCI as class IIB, II and III, respectively. Therefore, current guidelines recommend elective percutaneous therapy only if there are no other revascularization options; for example, cases in which surgical risk is too high, or when emergency intervention is needed, during angiography, because of hemodynamic instability [45, 46].

2.3
Data on Drug-eluting Stents in Unprotected Left Main Coronary Artery

The introduction of drug-eluting stents (DES) in clinical practice has significantly reduced the risk of restenosis and re-intervention thanks to the antiproliferative properties of the drug released. This has rapidly led to their widespread and extensive use, even for the treatment of more complex lesions that are considered off-label, such as ULMCA stenosis [47]. Many observational studies on patients with ULMCA disease have demonstrated the safety and efficacy of PCI with DES in a short- to medium-term follow-up, reporting a low mortality, ranging between 0% and 14% in low to high clinical risk patients, and a relatively low incidence of revascularization, ranging from 2% to 20% [48–61]. A recent meta-analysis of DES studies, with a medium-term follow-up (mean follow-up of 10 months), including a total of 1278 patients, reported an overall incidence of death, major cardiac events, and revascularization of 4.9%, 16.3%, and 6.6%, respectively [62]. More recently, observational registries of patients with ULMCA disease have confirmed these promising medium-term results of DES in the long term as well [63–68]. Most of the available data on medium- and long-term outcomes associated with the use of DES in the LMCA have been obtained from observational studies on populations treated with DES only; observational studies of DES versus BMS; and non-randomized studies of DES versus CABG. Only two randomized studies of DES versus CABG are currently available.

2.4
Observational Studies on Populations Treated with Drug-eluting Stents Only

All these studies have been consistent in showing favorable results in terms of safety and efficacy [48–52, 63–65]. Long-term outcomes of patients with ULMCA stenosis treated with DES have been reported in studies by Valgimigli et al., Tamburino et al., and Meliga et al. [63–65]. The former [63] assessed 55 patients treated with sirolimus-eluting stent (SES) and 55 treated with paclitaxel-eluting stent (PES) over a mean follow-up period of almost 2 years. The incidence of the composite of death or infarction and of target lesion revascularization (TLR) accounted for 16% and 9% in the SES group and 18% and 11% in the PES group, respectively [63]. The study by Tamburino et al. [64] reported on the outcomes of 210 patients over a mean period of more than 2 years. The cases studied showed an incidence of cardiac death and TLR of 4.3% and 8.2%, respectively. Most of the restenosis cases (91%) had a focal pattern, with an involvement of the left circumflex ostium alone [64]. Finally, the outcomes of patients who had undergone elective or emergency DES implantation to treat ULMCA lesions were assessed more extensively in 358 patients of the "DELFT" (Drug-Eluting stent for LeFT Main) registry [65], which reported the longest DES follow-up among those currently available in the literature. This study, including seven centers in Europe and the US, reported cardiac death and TLR incidences of 9.2% and 5.8%, respectively, at 3-year follow-up. The elective patients had a significantly lower risk of cardiac death during the follow-up compared to the emergency patients (6.2% vs. 21.4%; $P = 0.001$) [65]. DES studies, like the previous BMS studies, clearly show that there is a directly proportional relationship between the pre-procedure risk, correlated with the patient's clinical status, and mortality, which therefore in the majority of cases, is not directly ascribable to the procedure *per se*. It should be noted that in most of these studies the Euroscore was a strong independent predictor of mortality. Moreover, analysis with longer follow-up has shown that most of the adverse events occur during the first year and that the incidence of these events drops sharply and subsequently levels off, thus demonstrating an inversely proportional relationship between the length of follow-up and the incidence of adverse events, including stent thrombosis.

2.5
Observational Studies of Drug-eluting Stents Versus Bare Metal Stents

Registries comparing DES versus BMS in treating ULMCA disease have shown a drastic reduction in the risk of re-intervention associated with DES [53–57,

66]. These studies show that patients treated with DES tend to have more complex clinical and angiographic characteristics. However, this greater complexity in both patients and lesions treated with DES, is not associated with an increase in the incidence of death and myocardial infarction. Park et al. [54] reported 102 cases of patients with ULMCA disease treated electively with SES implantation, which were compared with 121 patients treated with BMS. After a 1-year follow-up patients treated with SES showed a significantly higher event-free survival compared to those of the BMS group (98 ± 1.4% vs. 81.4 ± 3.7; $P = 0.0003$), driven by a significantly lower incidence of TLR (2.0% in the SES group and 17.4% in the BMS group; $P < 0.001$). No case of death or myocardial infarction was reported over the follow-up. Follow-up angiography showed a restenosis rate of 7% in the SES group and 30.3% in the BMS group ($P < 0.001$); all restenoses in the SES group were located at the left main bifurcation. Similar results were reported by Chieffo et al. [55] in a study comparing a group of 85 patients with ULMCA lesions treated with DES with a historical group of 64 patients treated with BMS. After adjustment of data for the propensity score, at a 6-month follow-up, DES implantation proved to be associated with a lower risk of major adverse cardiac events (MACE) (odds ratio (OR), 0.27; 95% confidence interval (CI), 0.09 to 0.73; $P = 0.007$), TLR (OR, 0.28; 95% CI, 0.09 to 0.81; $P = 0.01$), and target vessel revascularization (TVR) (OR, 0.34; 95% CI, 0.12 to 0.91; $P = 0.03$). In this study as well, all restenoses in the DES group were focal and occurred at the left main bifurcation. The retrospective multi-center registry promoted by the Italian Society of Invasive Cardiology ("GISE-SICI [Gruppo Italiano Studi Emodinamici-Società Italiana di Cardiologia Invasiva] survey on ULMCA stenosis") is one of the largest studies on DES versus BMS, reporting outcomes of PCI performed on ULMCA lesions in 1453 patients, 1111 of whom were treated with DES (PES or SES) and 342 with BMS [66]. The risk of cardiac death over a 2-year follow-up, adjusted for the clinical and angiographic differences between the two groups, was significantly lower in the group undergoing DES, thus resulting in a 52% relative reduction in cardiac mortality. The benefit in reduced mortality associated with DES was especially significant in the 3- to 6-month period, during which the clinical effects of restenosis occurred, and it remained constant up to 2 years. In addition, the myocardial infarction and TLR incidence rates were both significantly lower in the group of DES patients. A sub-analysis [69] of this registry assessing 849 patients (58% of the registry's total population) with unstable angina or non-ST-segment elevation myocardial infarction (NSTEMI) (611 patients treated with DES and 238 with BMS) showed no significant reduction in 3-year overall mortality (adjusted hazard ratio (HR) 0.90; 95% CI 0.59–1.38; $P = 0.617$) and cardiac mortality (adjusted HR 0.75; 95% CI 0.45–1.27; $P = 0.287$) with DES. In contrast, the greater efficacy of DES compared to BMS was demonstrated in the reduction of the incidence of myocardial infarction (relative reduction of 63%, $P = 0.009$) and TLR (relative reduction of 62%, $P = 0.001$), over a 3-year follow-up [69]. A significant reduction in 3-year TLR risk, associated with DES compared to BMS (14.8% vs. 32.3%; $P = 0.001$, respectively; adjusted HR 0.33; 95% CI 0.14–0.80) was also confirmed in the subgroup of patients with diabetes in the GISE-SICI registry (a total of 398 patients, accounting for 28% of the registry's total population) [70]. The benefit of DES on TLR was not associated with a greater risk of death (adjusted HR 0.56; 95% CI 0.24–1.28) or myocardial infarction (adjusted HR 0.82; 95% CI 0.21–3.26) among patients with diabetes, who are well known for having a higher risk of thrombotic events compared to individuals without diabetes [70].

2.6
Non-randomized Studies of Drug-eluting Stents Versus Coronary Artery Bypass Grafting

The excellent results obtained with DES have suggested that these devices can be an effective and safe alternative to CABG when treating left main coronary artery disease, in cases with an anatomy that is suitable for percutaneous intervention. Several observational studies have reported short- and medium-term comparative data of PCI with DES versus CABG [58–61]. "The Bologna Registry" [58] is a prospective study on LMCA stenosis, comparing 154 patients treated surgically with 157 who underwent stenting. Of these, 94 received a DES. The two populations were quite homogeneous and differed only by mean age and surgical risk, which were both higher among patients treated with PCI, and by the incidence of acute coronary syndrome, which, by contrast, was higher among patients treated with CABG. During a mean follow-up of 14 months both overall and cardiac mortality did not differ between CABG and PCI (12% vs. 13% overall mortality and 9.7% vs. 9.5% cardiac mortality, respectively) and between CABG and DES (12% vs. 11.7% overall mortality and 9.7% vs. 7.4% cardiac mortality, respectively), even after the baseline clinical and angiographic differences between the two groups were adjusted for. By contrast, the need for revascularization was significantly higher in the PCI group (25.5% vs. 2.6%) [58]. Other comparative studies on CABG versus ULMCA PCI, among which, a smaller one evaluating 123 CABG patients and 50 DES patients [59], an Italian registry of 249 patients [60], of whom 107 were treated with DES, and a Spanish registry [61] including 96 patients receiving DES and 245 treated surgically, all reported medium-term results consistent with those of The Bologna Registry. ULMCA surgical and percutaneous treatment strategies were also compared in the subgroup of elderly patients [71, 72], who, despite improvements in surgical techniques and postoperative management, still have a high mortality and morbidity when treated surgically. An Italian registry [71] assessing the outcomes at 2 years following ULMCA treatment in 259 patients aged over 75 years, 161 of whom underwent CABG and 98 of whom received DES, showed no difference in the mortality rate (adjusted incidence of 15% vs. 13%, respectively, $P = 0.74$) and incidence of infarction (6% vs. 4%, respectively, $P = 0.88$). In the group of DES patients there was a higher incidence of TLR (25% vs. 3%, $P < 0.0001$). A recent study [72] has assessed 249 consecutive patients over 80 years of age: 145 underwent CABG and 104 PCI (48% received DES). The adjusted analysis of the baseline differences using the propensity score shows a similar survival rate free from cardiac death or infarction (PCI, 65.4%; CABG, 69.7%, adjusted HR 1.28; 95% CI, 0.64–2.56; $P = 0.47$), and free from major adverse cerebro-cardiovascular events (MACCE) (PCI, 56.7%; CABG, 64.8%; adjusted HR 1.11; 95% CI, 0.59–2.0; $P = 0.73$), during a mean follow-up of 23 $\pm$ 16 months.

Comparative data of CABG versus PCI in left main coronary artery disease with longer follow-up and larger patient populations are provided by the Korean multi-center registry "MAIN-COMPARE" [67]. In this study a total of 542 PCI patients were paired by clinical and angiographic characteristics with a corresponding group of patients treated with CABG. The same was done for patients receiving BMS and those receiving DES, thus obtaining 207 and 396 pairs of patients, respectively. There was no difference in mortality rate and in the composite incidence of death, infarction, or stroke, both when the entire group of PCI patients, regardless of the type of stent received, was compared to the CABG groups, and when the BMS and DES groups were considered and compared to the matching CABG group. By contrast, revascularization was significantly higher in the PCI group, among both the patients receiving BMS and those receiving DES. In another analysis of CABG versus PCI in ULMCA, there was no difference in 3-year mortality in 97 patients treated with PCI, paired, based on the propensity score, with a group of 190 CABG patients [68].

2.7
Randomized Studies of Drug-eluting Stents Versus Coronary Artery Bypass Grafting

Although DES registries have reported excellent results, reflecting hands-on experience in the "real world", and are essential in comparing the safety and efficacy of PCI versus CABG in the treatment of left main coronary artery stenosis, they have some intrinsic shortcomings due to selection bias and confounding factors that fail to be measured and adjusted even with sophisticated statistical adjustment and pairing techniques, thus affecting the results. This is why randomized trials are absolutely necessary for determining whether

PCI is as effective and safe as surgery. To date just one randomized study on CABG versus PCI for left main coronary artery disease (LE MANS, Unprotected Left Main Stenting Versus Bypass Surgery) has been published [73]. The trial compared the outcomes of patients with critical ULMCA disease undergoing PCI ($n = 52$) versus CABG ($n = 53$), with a mean follow-up of 28 months. The trial reported a similar incidence of adverse events at 2 years for both, with a better survival after stenting (71.2% vs. 75.5% in the PCI and CABG arms, respectively; $P = 0.29$) and a greater risk of re-intervention among patients undergoing angioplasty (relative risk (RR) 1.27; 95% CI 1.05–1.54; $P = 0.01$). However, DES was used only in 18 cases (35%), and high-risk patients, including those with acute infarction, a Euroscore >8, and renal failure, were excluded. The SYNTAX (Synergy between PCI with Taxus and Cardiac Surgery) trial results [74] were recently reported. Patients with left main coronary artery and/or three-vessel coronary artery disease were randomized for CABG ($n = 897$) or stenting with DES ($n = 903$) after an assessment of surgical risk and lesion complexity (quantified using the SYNTAX score) by an interventional cardiologist and cardiac surgeon. The primary endpoint was the composite incidence of death, myocardial infarction, cerebrovascular events, or any type of revascularization (PCI or CABG) at 1-year follow-up. The study population was also divided into subgroups depending on the extent of coronary artery disease: three-vessel coronary artery disease not involving LMCA (1,095 patients); coronary artery disease involving isolated LMCA (91 patients); or LMCA plus one (138 patients), two (218 patients), or three major coronary artery branches (258 patients). In all, left main coronary artery disease accounted for about 34% of patients, and primary endpoint incidence was similar in the CABG and PCI groups (13.7% vs. 15.8%; $P = 0.44$). An analysis of the subgroups showed that results tended to be better among CABG patients with left main coronary artery disease involving two (14.4% CABG vs. 19.8% PCI) or three (15.4% CABG vs. 19.3% PCI) vessels, while patients with isolated left main coronary artery disease (7.1% PCI vs. 8.5% CABG) and those who also have the involvement of a single vessel (7.5% PCI vs. 13.2% CABG) fare better with angioplasty. This suggests that patients with more extensive coronary artery disease and a higher SYNTAX score may gain greater benefit from surgical treatment. The SYNTAX score in our personal case history has proven to be reliable in distinguishing between patients with a high or low risk of mortality following left main angioplasty, with an optimal cut-off of 34. Data currently available in the literature suggest that PCI is a valid strategy that is as safe and effective as surgery, and that accurate selection of patients, lesions, and technique is the most important determinant of success.

2.8
Studies on the Prognostic Implications of Stenosis Location

Available data show that PCI is a safe and effective strategy for the treatment of left main coronary artery disease, with a reasonable incidence of both early and later adverse events. The main shortcoming is the relatively high percentage of restenoses affecting the bifurcation and, in particular, the left circumflex ostium, which some studies have correlated with the specific stenting technique applied. An analysis by Valgimigli et al. [75] on a subpopulation of patients in the RESEARCH (Rapamycin-Eluting Stent Evaluated At Rotterdam Cardiology Hospital) and T-SEARCH (Taxus-Stent Evaluated At Rotterdam Cardiology Hospital) registries receiving DES to treat ULMCA lesions showed that, in a median follow-up of 587 days, patients with a distal LMCA lesion had a higher incidence of cardiac events (30% vs. 11%: $P = 0.0007$) compared to patients with no distal LMCA involvement, principally because of higher incidence of revascularization of the target vessel (13% vs. 3%; $P = 0.02$). A sub-analysis of the DELFT registry [76] assessed the impact of lesion location and stenting technique on the outcomes and showed a greater incidence of TLR at 3 years in LMCA distal lesions treated with the implantation of two DES as opposed to those treated with a single stent. There was no difference in the overall incidence of cardiac events. A sub-analysis on the GISE-SICI survey [77] included 773 patients with a distal left main coronary artery lesion: 456 received a stent, while 317 received two stents. Over a 2-year follow-up, MACE-free survival (death, infarction, or TLR), adjusted for the baseline risk, was significantly higher among patients receiving a single stent compared to those receiving two stents (the propensity-adjusted HR for MACE risk in the single-stent versus two-stent group amounted to 0.53, 95% CI 0.37–0.76). This suggests that the stenting technique is an important prognostic factor. Therefore, the appropriate selection and optimization of bifurcation stenting technique are key to achieving and ensuring the success of the procedure in these high-risk lesions in the course of time. While there may still be some residual hesitation in treating stenoses with a distal location, which may be a factor limiting the long-term efficacy of PCI, it is now a matter of fact that the stenting of non-distal ULMCA lesions is a procedure with a high success rate, offering excellent medium- and long-term results in terms of safety and efficacy. A recent multi-center study that focused on 147 patients receiving DES (SES or PES stent) to treat non-distal ULMCA lesions (ostium and/or trunk) reported a low incidence of adverse cardiac events (7.4%) and restenosis (0.9%), with a follow-up of over 2 years [78].

2.9
Data on Drug-eluting Stents in Left Main Coronary Artery Trifurcation Lesions

The evolution of techniques and the use of DES has allowed interventional cardiologists to increasingly approach left main trifurcation lesions. However, only a few studies, including a small number of cases, have evaluated the safety and efficacy of DES implantation in this subset of lesions [79–82]. Furuichi et al. reported the outcomes in 13 patients after DES implantation in *de novo* distal left main trifurcation lesion. During a mean follow-up of 19 months, TLR occurred in 23.1% of cases. No deaths, Q-wave myocardial infarctions, or stent thromboses (ST) were recorded [79]. In a series of 20 patients with left main coronary artery trifurcation treated with DES, Shammas et al. reported a 29.4% rate of cumulative MACE (5.3% cardiac death) and 11.8% acute ST, during a median follow-up of about 9 months [80]. The largest experience of stenting for unprotected left main coronary artery trifurcation disease was reported by Sheiban et al. [81]. A MACE rate of 33% (cardiac death 15% and myocardial infarction 4%) and definite ST rate of 3% were recorded, in a total of 27 patients at long-term follow-up (median 28 months) [81]. Finally, in a series of 11 patients with clinically significant *de novo* left main coronary artery trifurcation lesion, Tamburino et al. observed a 27% incidence of TLR and 9% incidence of cardiac death, at 24 months of mean follow-up [82]. Overall, these results are consistent in showing that stenting of this subset of high-risk lesions is feasible and is associated with an acceptable incidence of TLR and favorable safety results, considering the complexity of lesions and patients treated.. Nonetheless, larger studies with longer follow-up are needed to confirm these promising results.

2.10
Final Considerations Based on Available Data

1. Percutaneous treatment of ULMCA stenosis is a technically feasible strategy associated with a high procedural success rate and is quite simple to perform for interventional cardiologists with consistent experience in this specific subgroup of "challenging lesions".
2. Drug-eluting stents have made it possible to achieve excellent results in terms of medium- and long-term safety, with results that are as good as those obtained with CABG. The various studies show no difference in mortality and myocardial infarction rates between CABG and PCI using DES.
3. It has been widely demonstrated that these safety endpoints are affected by pre-procedure baseline clinical risk (clinical presentation, comorbidities, etc)

rather than by the revascularization procedure *per se*. "Patient selection" is thus a determinant with regard to mortality in the acute phase and at follow-up.

4. Drug-eluting stents are associated with excellent results in terms of efficacy and the need for re-intervention in the follow-up. Nonetheless, studies show that TVR/TLR incidence is higher compared to CABG. However, the higher risk of undergoing another PCI in the follow-up needs to be offset against the high risk of morbidity associated with CABG, prompting patients to prefer a non-invasive strategy, which, while not associated with an increase in mortality, has the potential of improving the quality of survival.

5. It has been demonstrated that in the vast majority of cases, re-intervention on the target lesion is due to restenosis (usually with a "focal" pattern) at the bifurcation and, more precisely, at the left circumflex ostium. It appears that this endpoint is greatly affected by factors related to technique and procedure. Optimization of the procedure and technique for bifurcation stenting may narrow the gap between CABG and PCI. "Proper lesion and technique selection" are determinants for restenosis.

6. The overall incidence of adverse events appears to be rather low after 1 year, suggesting that close clinical and angiographic monitoring, along with optimal antiplatelet regimes, are especially important only during the first 12 months following the procedure.

7. More recent data show that PCI has slightly less favorable outcomes compared to CABG in cases of diffuse and complex multi-vessel coronary artery disease. The reason seems to be the difficulty in achieving optimal and complete percutaneous revascularization of the lesions outside the left main coronary artery compared to revascularization of the co-existent left main coronary artery lesion.

Morpho-functional Assessment of Left Main Coronary Artery Disease

3

3.1
Introduction

The morpho-functional assessment of LMCA stenoses plays an essential role both in therapeutic decision making and in the assessment of post-PCI results. While still being considered the gold standard method in the diagnosis of LMCA stenosis, conventional coronary angiography shows all its shortcomings in the quantitative assessment of those lesions, as proven in several studies confirming a high degree of interobserver variability [83–85]. These shortcomings are especially relevant in the case of the LMCA, as the severity of the stenosis correlates with the clinical outcome of patients, and a degree of angiographic stenosis of over 50% is acknowledged as the cut-off for treatment [86]. Moreover, simple angiographic assessment after stent implantation may not ensure a good final result in terms of stent expansion, with the ensuing risk of adverse events such as in-stent thrombosis.

For this reason, angiography often needs to be associated with other conventional invasive assessment techniques both of a morphological nature like intravascular ultrasound (IVUS), and of a functional nature like pressure gradient measurement (fractional flow reserve, FFR). Alongside these techniques, other more recent ones like three-dimensional (3D) quantitative coronary analysis (QCA) are proposed as additional methods that are useful in the assessment of LMCA stenosis. It is likely that in the future, the use of other techniques such as optical coherence tomography (OCT) will gain ground in the study of these lesions.

In addition, besides invasive methods, new non-invasive imaging techniques such as multi-slice computed tomography (MSCT) and cardiovascular magnetic resonance (CMR) have recently been introduced into clinical practice and they are set to become useful tools in the morphological and functional assessment of atherosclerotic disease both during the diagnostic phase and in the post-procedure follow-up.

This is not the place for a detailed description of the single methods, as the purpose of this text is limited to the clinical application of these techniques in LMCA disease.

3.2
The Role of Intravascular Ultrasound

Although the literature lacks data from randomized clinical studies on the usefulness of IVUS in the era of DES, it is definitely a useful technique and, at times, it is absolutely necessary both for an adequate diagnosis of LMCA atherosclerotic disease and as a guide for the PCI revascularization procedure. In fact, it provides more quantitative and qualitative information than angiography alone, thus offering better guidance in therapeutic decision making (Fig. 3.1). It has recently been demonstrated, among other things, that the use of IVUS during DES implantation in various coronary artery segments including the LMCA is associated with a lower rate of in-stent thrombosis, and there seems to be a trend towards a lower rate of restenosis [87].

LMCA lesions, compared to other coronary artery lesions, have peculiar features that often require clinicians to perform intracoronary ultrasound.

In order to fully grasp the diagnostic potential of IVUS, various scenarios illustrating the typical limits of angiography need to be considered:
• angiography often underestimates the severity of LMCA lesions
• at times it is difficult to angiographically determine the reference diameter when the LMCA is diffusely diseased; this can lead to the choice of an incorrect stent diameter, thus negatively impacting the outcome of PCI
• at times the rebound to contrast injection in the aortic bulb does not allow a proper visualization of the LMCA ostium
• LMCA with acute aortic take-off and a curve along the shaft is often mistaken for critical stenosis at angiography
• in cases of distal LMCA disease, IVUS affords a full understanding of the involvement of the bifurcation's carina and the side branch ostium
• angiography provides general information on plaque composition (degree of calcification) and the presence of ulcers and/or dissections (Fig. 3.2).

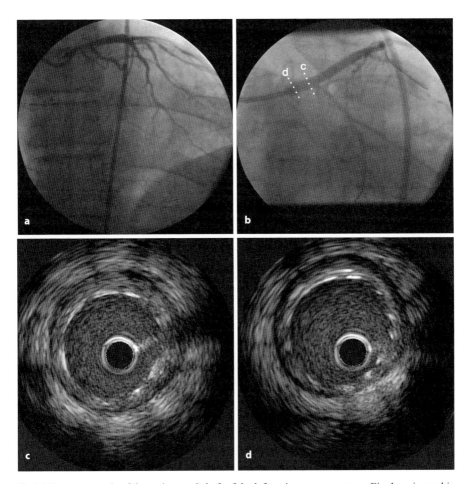

Fig. 3.1 Severe stenosis of the ostium and shaft of the left main coronary artery. Final angiographic result after implantation of 3.5/13 mm Cypher stent (**b**); *dotted lines* correspond to IVUS scan planes as shown in **c** and **d** respectively. IVUS images at the distal (**c**) and proximal segments (**d**) of the stent confirm the good final angiographic result

Although the literature does not offer homogeneous data on the IVUS criteria and on the corresponding cut-off values to define critical LMCA stenosis, there is widespread consensus in recommending LMCA revascularization with a minimal lumen diameter (MLD) of <2.8 mm and a minimum lumen area

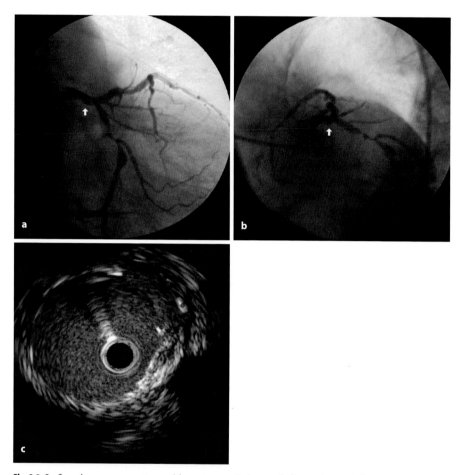

Fig. 3.2 Left main coronary artery with a suspected ulcerated plaque (*arrows*) in caudal posterior-anterior (**a**) and caudal left anterior oblique views (**b**). IVUS image confirms the presence of plaque ulceration (*red points*) without significant stenosis (**c**)

(MLA) of <6 mm². This parameter is the result of Murray's law [88] and of a study by Jasti et al. who correlated IVUS with the FFR [89]. The application of these parameters makes it possible to identify critical lesions with a high degree of accuracy and to exclude angiographic false positives.

In cases of diffuse disease or a short LMCA, the lack of a lesion-free section hinders the proper assessment of the reference diameter. Clearly, this problem can be bypassed by using IVUS, as it provides detailed information on the actual dimensions of the LMCA, thus allowing the right device to be chosen.

Qualitative information on the composition of the atherosclerotic plaque is just as important; medial and intimal calcification arcs with angles >180° may require debulking to optimize DES implantation.

Finally, in the assessment of distal LMCA the use of IVUS is now considered a must. Not only it is useful in optimizing PCI following DES implantation by offering guidance in the choice of the balloon for post-dilation, but it is also extremely valuable in accurately determining the distribution of atherosclerotic disease in the bifurcation's segments, thus facilitating the choice of the most appropriate percutaneous technique (see Chapter 4).

Data in the literature on the use of IVUS guidance for PCI of LMCA with DES [90, 91] show that the use of IVUS seems to be associated with a reduction in 3-year mortality and that a final minimum stent area (MSA) of >8.5 mm^2 reduces TLR to the minimum.

3.3
Procedure for Performing Intravascular Ultrasound in the Left Main Coronary Artery

The procedure for performing IVUS in the LMCA does not differ from that used in other vessels. However, some technical features need to be taken into account.

- Automatic pull-back at a rate of 0.5 mm/s is the technique adopted. If the LMCA is very long, the pull-back speed can be set at 1 mm/s to reduce the examination's execution time, and hence limit ischemia due to the ultrasound probe.
- In cases of tight lesions, the intracoronary probe may occlude the left main coronary artery, thus leading to hemodynamic instability in the patient; in these cases it is recommended to perform the IVUS run after dilatation with a small-diameter balloon (2.0–2.5 mm).
- JL4 guiding catheters are recommended, as they avoid deep intubation of the LMCA in order to thoroughly examine its entire course.
- After positioning the intracoronary guidewire and the IVUS probe, it is quite useful to decannulate the guiding catheter from the LMCA to better assess the ostium.
- The guiding catheter's tip should be oriented co-axially, especially in the case of a LMCA vessel with a large diameter, in order to study every layer of the vessel wall.

- Shortly before the start of the run, the image's depth should be increased to the maximum because of the LMCA's dimensions compared to other vessels.
- When examining the bifurcation, double wiring through both branches of the bifurcation is very useful, not only to protect the daughter vessels' ostia, but also to reduce the bifurcation angle for a better assessment of the side branch's carina and ostium; moreover, a left circumflex guidewire is a useful ultrasound point of reference in case of early diagonal or marginal branches, which may cause confusion in interpreting the images.

3.4
The Role of Fractional Flow Reserve

FFR is a severity index for coronary artery stenosis that expresses the maximum flow achievable in a coronary artery as a fraction of the maximum blood flow, which is normally obtained in the same area of the myocardium of a healthy subject [92].

Measuring the FFR makes it possible to perform a functional assessment of the ability of a coronary artery stenosis to induce ischemia both at rest and during pharmacological stress. Many studies have proven the usefulness of this method in the prognostic assessment of angiographically intermediate stenoses present in the various coronary artery segments and shown that a value of FFR ≥0.75 is favorably correlated with the clinical outcome in patients receiving medical therapy [93–95]. The application of FFR in LMCA lesions has been assessed in small clinical trials, which have all confirmed the results already achieved in other coronary artery segments [89, 96–100]. While data in the literature on the role of FFR in LMCA stenoses are homogeneous, nonetheless it should be borne in mind that these trials have evident shortcomings in terms of both the number and type of patients enrolled, and that these cannot be extended to all subgroups of patients affected by LMCA disease such as, for instance, those with diabetes or with a low left ventricular ejection fraction (LVEF) among whom other factors may contribute to the prognosis.

FFR can be applied with benefit in PCI treatment of the LMCA. The potential for mapping the entire coronary arterial tree makes it possible, for instance, to determine – in patients with multi-vessel disease affecting the LMCA – which stenoses are actually critical, and hence to selectively guide treatment during PCI [94]. Furthermore, for diagnostic purposes, FFR measurement can also be used intra-procedurally when treating LMCA bifurcation percutaneously, in order to assess the need for provisional stenting of the side branch or for complex stenting owing to the presence of residual stenosis of the branch following LMCA stenting [101].

In practical terms, specific expedients must be taken into account to perform an accurate measurement of the FFR in the LMCA:

- continuous intravenous administration of adenosine or other vasopressor agents is to be preferred over intracoronary bolus
- decannulate the guide catheter from the left main coronary artery's ostium while measuring the pressure
- slowly perform the pull-back of the pressure guidewire
- measure the FFR in both the LAD and the LCX.

Contrary to IVUS, for which there is no consensus on the optimal cut-off to define critical stenosis of the LMCA, all the studies performed on FFR measurement agree in setting an FFR value of 0.75 as the optimal cut-off. Considering that the current guidelines recommend that myocardial revascularization, either percutaneous or surgical, should be performed only once inducible ischemia in that given area has been proven and, considering the aforementioned limits of conventional angiography, there is a clear prognostic benefit resulting from the "test" on suspected LMCA ischemia using FFR, as demonstrated by the various studies published. This can avoid inappropriate treatment, either percutaneously or surgically, of patients with subcritical LMCA disease.

3.5
The Role of Optical Coherence Tomography

OCT is an invasive imaging technique recently introduced into clinical practice. It is based on real-time tomographic image reconstruction from backscattered reflections of infrared light. Thanks to its high spatial longitudinal resolution of around 10–15 μm, it allows the *in vivo* morphological study of atherosclerotic plaque with microscopic resolution. Several studies have demonstrated that OCT can be used to examine the various plaque components (lipid pool, calcifications, thrombus, etc) during its various stages of development (stable, unstable, ulcered, etc). It also offers the possibility of documenting the presence of thin-cap fibroatheroma or cellular elements like macrophages, which are a typical marker of vulnerability [102]. Besides for the morphological study of the plaque, OCT has also been proposed for the study of DES re-endothelialization and the correlated pathological phenomena such as the long-term persistence of uncovered stent struts, which are believed to be the possible triggers of in-stent thrombosis [103]. Moreover, like IVUS, OCT makes it possible to measure various vessel geometry parameters such as MLD, MLA, and MSA. These provide useful information on the extent of the stenosis and the post-stenting result.

However, the OCT systems currently available in clinical practice (LightLab M2 and M3 systems) have technical limits. These include the poor penetration of infrared light into blood and tissues, which makes it impossible to examine vessel walls thicker than 1.5 mm; the need to exclude blood by flushing with an isotonic solution after proximal occlusion, or with a hypo-osmolar contrast agent (iodixanol) without balloon occlusion; and the slowness of pull-back (2–3 mm/s depending on the version). These reasons probably also explain why there are currently no trials specifically assessing the use of OCT in the assessment of LMCA disease, since the diameter of this vessel, especially after stenting, does not make it possible to obtain good-quality images.

In practice, when performing OCT of the LMCA, some expedients are needed:
• image acquisition must be performed with the non-occlusive technique by flushing with hypo-osmolar contrast agent (proximal occlusion with the balloon is not possible in the LMCA)
• position the tip of the guide catheter at the ostium of the LMCA before pull-back allowing flushing and scanning of the body and bifurcation segments of the vessel
• perform the pull-back both from the LCX and from the LAD to examine the LMCA's bifurcation.

A new version of the OCT system with fast pull-back (Optical Frequency Domain Imaging, OFDI) is currently being clinically validated [104] and it seems that it will be able to make up for the limitations of the first generation in the study of LMCA disease.

3.6
Three-dimensional Quantitative Coronary Analysis Reconstruction of the Left Main Coronary Artery

Despite the great advances made in recent years in non-invasive cardiovascular imaging and the introduction of powerful instruments such as multi-slice computerized tomography (MSCT) scan, positron emission tomography (PET), and magnetic resonance imaging (cardiovascular magnetic resonance, CMR), conventional coronary angiography is still the gold standard for the assessment of epicardial coronary artery disease. The complex and actual geometry of the coronary arterial tree can be reconstructed through the acquisition of two-dimensional (2D) images from different views.

Depending on the views used and/or partial vascular overlapping that may occur in 2D imaging, errors may occur, however, in the assessment of the actual length of coronary artery branches, their diameter, and the presence and severity of stenosis. In addition to this, it is impossible to fully appreciate the main anatomical features of the coronary arterial tree in a 2D image, such as vessel curvature and the take-off angles at the bifurcation, which are essential in the study of the hemodynamic factors linked to atherosclerosis and for the choice of the interventional approach to treat any lesions [105, 106].

The LMCA is one of the segments of the coronary arterial tree that are most difficult to assess angiographically (direct origin from aorta, shortness, variable course, stenosing disease, at times either diffuse or eccentric, etc). The absence of fixed anchorage to surrounding structures and extensive atherosclerotic involvement of the vessel's wall can lead to underestimation of the disease. An abnormal origin or spasm of the LMCA, the presence of aortic valve stenosis, the injection of an inadequate amount of contrast agent or at too slow a rate leading to inadequate vessel filling can also lead to a poor assessment of the disease [107].

3D coronary reconstructions make it possible to accurately define the extent, complexity, and length of the lesion, the degree of stenosis, and the reference vessel diameter (RVD), thus allowing a thorough and appropriate assessment of the indication for interventional treatment, and offering guidance in the selection of the most appropriate material [108–111].

The 3D model obtained can also be freely rotated in space, thus making it possible to analyze the vessels from different viewpoints and to assess both the LMCA and the bifurcation's side branch as well as the take-off angles.

There are various 3D coronary artery modeling systems based on 2D angiography images. CardioOp-B and Philips Allura Integris are the software systems currently available (Fig. 3.3). Coronary artery morphology is described with a high level of accuracy: minimal lumen diameter ±0.14 mm, lesion length ±2.4 mm and minimal lumen area ±0.31 mm^2. 3D image processing takes 4 to 30 minutes (Fig. 3.4) [112].

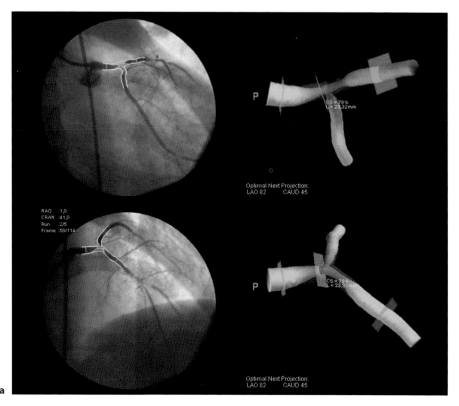

a

Fig. 3.3 (*cont.⟶*)

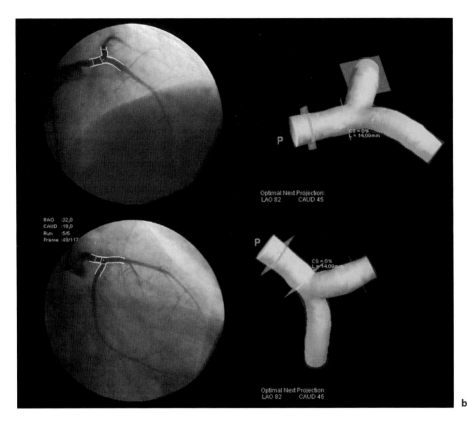

Fig. 3.3 (*cont.*) Angiographic images of severe distal LMCA stenosis involving the LAD and LCX (*left panel*) with corresponding 3D reconstruction (*right panel*), before (**a**) and after (**b**) stenting, from the integration of two single-plane angiographic images taken from different angles.

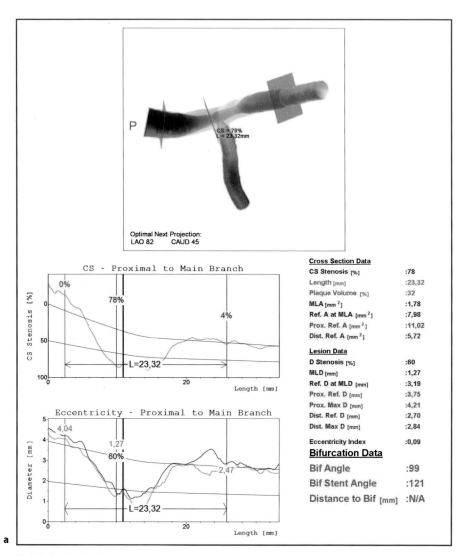

Fig. 3.4 (*cont.*———►)

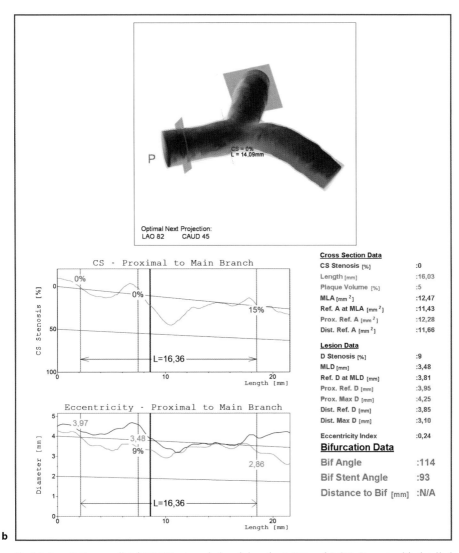

b

Fig. 3.4 (*cont.*) Severe distal LMCA stenosis involving the LAD and LCX. Report with detailed data regarding lesion scenarios, bifurcation main- and side-branch geometry, cross-section area, and eccentricity graphs before (**a**) and after (**b**) stenting

3.7
The Role of Multi-slice Computed Tomography

In recent years MSCT has seen rapid technological development, which has allowed this technique to establish itself as a possible non-invasive alternative to conventional coronary angiography in diagnosing atherosclerotic coronary artery disease [113]. Latest-generation 64-slice scanners have dramatically improved the diagnostic performance of coronary computed tomographic angiography (CCTA) compared to previous 16-slice versions, and continual improvements are being made in reducing the still significantly high doses of radiation [114]. Recently, a multi-center prospective randomized study has assessed 64-slice CCTA compared to conventional coronary angiography, including 230 subjects with chest pain and an intermediate risk of coronary artery disease (CAD), and its results are of great clinical interest: in the analysis per patient, CCTA sensitivity and specificity compared to coronary angiography in diagnosing stenosis of ≥50% and ≥70% was 95% and 83%, and 94% and 83%, respectively, while the negative predictive value was 99% [115].

LMCA assessment via CCTA is especially convenient, as the vessel generally has a large diameter, its course runs axially compared to the scanning direction, and it is relatively stable, thus making it less susceptible to movement artifacts. In fact, CCTA has proven to be especially effective in assessing LMCA disease compared to both coronary angiography [116] and IVUS [117], showing a sensitivity and specificity of 100% in both cases.

One recently published study using 40-slice MSCT has assessed the distribution of atherosclerotic plaque at LMCA bifurcation, showing that it is located mainly at the LAD ostium and in a position opposite the LAD flow divider, and also showing how the LMCA bifurcation angle correlates with disease, which occurs most frequently at angles ≥88.5° [118].

Another interesting application of CCTA lies in the follow-up assessment of LMCA treatment with DES. A prospective study assessed 70 patients receiving DES to treat LMCA, using a 16-slice scanner (27 patients) and a 64-slice scanner (43 patients) at a mean interval of 259 days. These were then compared with the results from coronary angiography and IVUS. Overall diagnostic accuracy amounted to 93% in identifying angiographic in-stent restenosis (ISR), which, however, rose to 98% if stenting was extended to one of the main branches, while it dropped to 83% in cases of complex bifurcation stenting. Sensitivity and specificity were to 100% and 91%, respectively. CCTA correlation with IVUS was good ($r = 0.78$ and 0.73, respectively), with an IVUS threshold of ≥1 mm to identify ISR via CCTA [119].

MSCT can also be used for the morphological assessment of LMCA disease as demonstrated for other coronary artery segments [120] (Fig. 3.5).

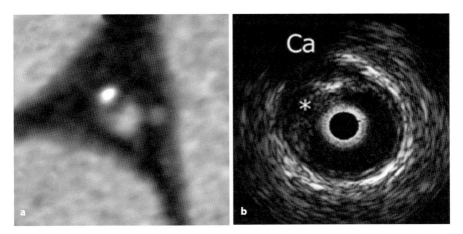

Fig. 3.5 A cross-section of a left main coronary artery with an eccentric atherosclerotic lesion characterized by mixed components visualized on CT (**a**) and IVUS (**b**). There is an external calcification (*Ca* in **b**) and internal non-calcified layer (*asterisk*). Supplied courtesy of Dr. Filippo Cademartiri, Dr. Francesca Pugliese, Dr. Gaston Rodriguez-Granillo, and Dr. Pim J De Feyter; Department of Radiology and Cardiology, Erasmus Medical Center, Rotterdam, The Netherlands

3.8
The Role of Cardiovascular Magnetic Resonance

Over the past decade, CMR has developed to become a potential non-invasive alternative to conventional coronary angiography in diagnosing atherosclerotic coronary artery disease and avoiding exposure to ionizing radiations and the administration of iodinated contrast agent. Moreover, the wide range of available sequences makes CMR suitable for the morphological study of atherosclerotic plaque [121]. However, the study of coronary arteries with CMR is made technically cumbersome owing to various factors such as the small diameter of vessels and their tortuous course, the signal from epicardial fat and the myocardium, the constant movement linked to cardiac and respiratory cycles, and the time limits due to the short data-recording interval during diastole when the flow through coronary arteries is greater. From this point of view and owing to its anatomical features, LMCA is one of the coronary artery segments that can be best visualized and studied with coronary magnetic resonance angiography (CMRA) (Fig. 3.6). In fact, in the only international multi-center trial hitherto published, Kim et al. used free-breathing 3D CMRA on 109 patients before elective conventional coronary angiography, and demonstrated in the per-segment analysis that 88% of LMCA cases could be interpreted to identify

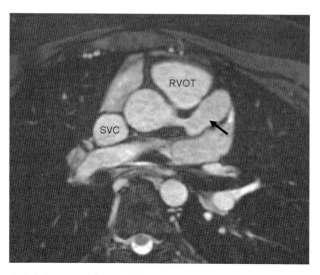

Fig. 3.6 A trans-axial magnetic resonance image acquired using a diaphragmatic navigator showing a large aneurysm of the left main coronary artery (*arrow*) of a young man with Kawasaki disease. *SVC*: superior vena cava; *RVOT*: right ventricular outflow tract. Supplied courtesy of Dr. Sanjay K. Prasad, Cardiovascular Magnetic Resonance Unit, Royal Brompton Hospital, London, UK

stenosis >50%, with a diagnostic accuracy of 89% and a negative predictive value of 98%. They concluded that this technique reliably identifies LMCA disease [122]. These results were recently confirmed by Sakuma et al. who applied a new whole-heart 3D CMRA technique and confirmed its usefulness on 131 patients in a prospective study in which the per-segment analysis showed a negative predictive value of 100% and a diagnostic accuracy of 98% in LMCA assessment [123].

At CMR, coronary artery stents appear like areas of signal void because of the metal. This technique makes it impossible to accurately perform a follow-up assessment of ISR in the LMCA.

While further technological progress is needed to allow CMRA to replace other invasive techniques that are not based on the use of X-rays for the study of the entire coronary arterial tree, CMRA does seem to be useful in assessing selected patients with suspect LMCA disease, and in their follow-up.

Left Main Coronary Artery Percutaneous Interventions: Materials and Techniques

4

4.1 Introduction

Before discussing this topic in more detail, a series of general considerations needs to be made:
- not all LMCA lesions should be treated with PCI
- LMCA lesions can be easily treated without major concerns in experienced centers by skilled and experienced operators
- the success of LMCA PCI depends on the availability of material and devices and the use of an appropriate technique
- in all LMCA lesions, pre-dilatation provides sufficient blood flow inside the main left coronary artery
- on the other hand, a tight lesion allows a stable stent positioning, especially at an ostial or shaft location
- when treating bifurcations, temporary occlusion of the LMCA, LAD, and LCX during use of a kissing balloon does not jeopardize the procedure
- the learning curve is crucial in choosing the best option for each case, after guiding catheter positioning.

Left Main Coronary Artery Disease, C. Tamburino.
© Springer-Verlag Italia 2009

4.2
Materials

4.2.1
Guiding Catheters

Despite the anatomic variability, almost all LMCAs can be easily cannulated by Judkins left, XB left, and left Amplatz guiding catheters. A 7 or 8 Fr size is recommended, especially if lesion preparation (rotablator, thrombus aspiration) or triple kissing balloon is scheduled. The availability of arterial closure or sealing systems allows the use of ≥7 Fr catheters, which are to be preferred. In case of difficult anatomy, emergent or complicated procedure (stent loss/entrapment, distal dissection, acute thrombosis), a larger catheter provides better maneuverability, dye injection, and device trackability. This is especially true when IVUS is needed.

In the case of a tortuous, long, and enlarged aorta, a long, metal reinforced sheath (Super Arrow Flex, 45, 65, 80, 100 cm), provides a strong and stable back-up, with greater maneuverability and stabilization of the guiding catheter. When ostial stent implantation is planned, it is possible to perform maneuvers or use systems that allow the interventionalist to accurately identify the LMCA ostium and carry out optimal stent deployment, avoiding stent hang-out [124, 125]. Side-hole guiding catheters are responsible for a high amount of dye injection, but allow a safe procedure without dumping pressure.

4.2.2
Coronary Wires

Tables 4.1 and 4.2 show the coronary wires most frequently used in LMCA PCI. In general, a soft-tipped spring wire (BMW or similar) is most commonly used

Table 4.1 Soft-tipped spring wires

Manufacturer	Wire	Diameter tip (inches) and stiffness (g)	Coating characteristics
Abbott Vascular	BMW, BMW Universal	0.014, 1	Non-hydrophilic
Asahi Intec	Prowater flex	0.014, 1	Non-hydrophilic
Terumo	Runthrough NS floppy	0.014, 1	Hydrophilic
	Runthrough NS hypercoat	0.014, 1	Hyper-hydrophilic

Table 4.2 Soft-medium tipped plastic wires

Manufacturer	Wire	Diameter tip (inches) and stiffness (g)	Coating characteristics	Spring at the tip
Boston Scientific	Choice PT2	0.014, 2	Polymer-hydrophilic	No
Abbott Vascular	Pilot 50, 150, 200	0.014, 2–5	Polymer-hydrophilic	Yes
Cordis J&J	Shinobi	0.014, 2	Polymer-hydrophilic	Yes
	Shinobi plus	0.014, 4	Polymer-hydrophilic	Yes
Terumo	Crosswire NT	0.014, 5.5	Polymer-hydrophilic	No

in LMCA percutaneous treatment. The vessel's vicinity to the aorta and its large diameter make lesion crossing easier thanks to this guidewire, whose main feature is that it provides moderate support with excellent flexibility. In the presence of major vessel calcification, excessive winding, extremely acute angles between the LMCA and LAD or LCX, lesion eccentricity, or ulcerated plaque at risk of destabilization, a hydrophilic guidewire (but best medium tipped) is more indicated and hence recommended, as it reaches the periphery with greater ease while providing greater support during the procedure.

4.2.3
Coronary Balloons

In order to prepare the lesion when conditions do not allow direct stenting (e.g. in the case of bifurcation lesion, calcified or severe lesion, eccentric plaque, etc), pre-dilatation with compliant or semi-compliant balloons is indicated (Table 4.3). Not only does pre-dilatation allow accurate lesion appraisal, but it facilitates the subsequent complete expansion of the stent and hence proper placement on the vessel wall. This appears to reduce the likelihood of occurrence of the much-feared event of subacute stent thrombosis, which, fortunately, is very rare in the case of LMCA-PCI and seems to be linked also to stent underexpansion, especially in the case of DES implantation [126, 127].

Once the stent is placed, post-dilatation with non-compliant balloons expanded to medium pressure (mandatory when treating bifurcation lesions) is recommended in the great majority of cases. Current evidence supports the need for stent post-dilatation in order to optimize stent deployment and assure a better outcome in terms of lower incidence of stent thrombosis and TVR at follow-up [128–131] (Tables 4.3, 4.4).

Table 4.3 Compliant balloons

Manufacturer	Balloon	Shaft length (cm) and diameter (Fr)	Balloon size (diameter × length), mm,	Entry tip profile, inches	Balloon crossing profile, inches
Cordis	Firestar	145, 1.9–2.7	2.50–4.00 × 8–30	0.014	0.025
Terumo	Rujin plus	145, 2.4–2.6	1.25–5.0 × 10–15–20	0.016	0.023
Boston	Maverick	140, 1.8–2.7	2.50–4.00 × 2.5–30	0.017	0.023
Abbott	Voyager	143, 2.4–2.7	2.5–4.00 × 8–30	0.017	0.024
	Mercury	140–145, 2.0–2.7	2.50–4.50 × 11–20	0.017	0.028
Medtronic	Sprinter	138, 1.9–2.4	2.5–5.00 × 6–30	0.017	0.024

Table 4.4 Non-compliant balloonss

Manufacturer	Balloon	Shaft length (cm) and diameter (Fr)	Balloon size (diameter × length), mm,	Nominal pressure, atmospheres	Rated burst pressure atmospheres
Cordis	Durastar	145, 2.7–1.9	2.25–4.0 × 10–15–20–25–30	14	20
Terumo	Hiyru	145, 2.6–2.0	2.25–5.0 × 6–14–16–20	10	20
Boston	Quantum	145, 1.8–2.7	2.0–5.0 × 8–10–12–15–20–30	12	20
SIS Medical AG	OPN NC	140, 2.45–1.9	2.0–4.0 × 10–15–20	12	32

4.2.4
Coronary Stents

Tables 4.5 and 4.6 show the stents commonly used in LMCA treatment. Several studies comparing BMS and DES in LMCA treatment confirm a general superiority of DES in terms of medium-/long-term MACE, above all, due to lower ISR and hence TVR incidence [54–57, 66, 69, 70]. The advantage of the use of

Table 4.5 Drug-eluting stents: dilatation limit after post-dilatation with non-compliant, low-profile, high-pressure balloon

Manufacturer	DES	Nominal stent diameter (mm)	Maximum post-dilatation stent diameter (mm)
Cordis	Cypher Select™ +	3.00	3.50
		3.50	4.50
Boston Scientific	Taxus™ Liberté™	3.00	4.25
		3.50	4.25
		4.00	5.75
		4.50	5.75
		5.00	5.75
Medtronic	Endeavor Resolute	3.00	3.50
		3.50	4.00
		4.00	4.50
Abbott	Xience V	3.00	3.50
		3.50	4.50
		4.00	4.50
Terumo	Nobori	3.00	3.50
		3.50	4.50

Table 4.6 Bare metal stent dilatation limit after post-dilatation with non-compliant, low-profile, high-pressure balloon

Manufacturer	BMS	Nominal stent diameter (mm)	Maximum post-dilatation stent diameter (mm)
Medtronic	Driver and Micro-Driver	3.00	5.00
		3.50	5.00
		4.00	5.00
		4.50	5.00
Abbott	Multi-link Vision	3.00	3.75
		3.50	4.50
		4.00	4.50

Table 4.7 Stent dilatation limit after post-dilatation with non-compliant, low-profile, high-pressure balloon: Catania™ stent, cobalt chromium stent with surface treatment by nanothin polyzene-F-non-trombogenic polymer

Manufacturer	Stent	Nominal stent diameter (mm)	Max post- dilatation stent diameter (mm)
Celonova	Catania™	3.00	3.50
		3.50	4.50
		4.00	4.50

DES over BMS is that they are narrower in less complex lesions, such as those located in the ostium and shaft. The LMCA's anatomical features (large RVD >3.00 mm and length of the segment to be stented of no more than 20 mm) seem to reduce TVR incidence in this subset of lesions, and hence afford an advantage of DES use over BMS. Few studies are currently available in the literature to support this theory. A recent paper [78] reported experience with 144 patients with diseased ostium and shaft, undergoing DES. It showed a favorable short- and medium-term outcome, in particular, in terms of TVR incidence. However, the data of the multi-center registry of the Società Italiana di Cardiologia Invasiva (Italian Society of Invasive Cardiology) (SICI-GISE) have made the greatest contribution in this regard. The outcome in patients receiving BMS or DES overlapped in terms of TVR [13]. However, randomized trials are needed in order to confirm this hypothesis (Tables 4.5, 4.6).

When discussing stents, it should be borne in mind that every model has a maximum achievable diameter. When treating a large-sized LMCA, it is recommended to use stents that can be over-expanded at high pressures, taking care of the maximum possible diameter per stent (Tables 4.5, 4.6 and 4.7), or stents that are used in other non-coronary arterial segments (renal stents) can even be used.

Moreover, it is necessary to consider that every segment of the LMCA requires specific treatment because of the different anatomical and functional characteristics of each. Therefore, specific and distinct therapeutic approaches are necessary for LMCA ostium, shaft, and bifurcation lesions.

4.3
Ostial Lesions

LMCA ostial lesions (Fig. 4.1) are commonly considered to be technically challenging. In order to ensure simple, effective, and safe percutaneous treatment of LMCA ostial lesions, the following aspects need to be taken into account:

- the LMCA ostium is composed mainly of elastic fibers. This feature accounts for the greater risk of elastic recoil and explains why the result of the procedure has improved with the introduction of stents in the percutaneous treatment of this lesion [133]
- the normal oscillation of the guiding catheter, especially in elderly patients with a dilated sclerotic aorta and high differential blood pressure, increases the risk of stent malpositioning (hang-out or ostial missing)
- the take-off of the LMCA from the aorta may require specific technical expedients and the use of specific guiding catheters to ensure adequate support while favoring optimal ostial stent positioning
- ostial stenosis in a short LMCA may require treatment of the vessel up to the bifurcation; in this case a main across side strategy is generally adopted
- the size of the LMCA may be large and hence require stents with a larger diameter not commonly used in coronary arteries (e.g. renal stents), as coronary stents with a diameter greater than 5.0 mm are not currently available on the market.

Having said this, and adopting the solutions needed for the various anatomical situations, the percutaneous treatment of the LMCA ostium can be consid-

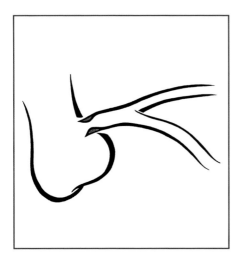

Fig. 4.1 Ostial lesion

ered a relatively simple procedure with a low risk of relapse throughout the follow-up [78, 132]. Once the LMCA is cannulated with a guiding catheter providing adequate support, the following maneuvers can be performed to achieve optimal stent placement:

- place the coronary guidewire at the tip of the LAD trying to obtain a distal loop. By further advancing the guidewire, this allows a retrograde catheter movement, without any risk of distal perforation. This makes it possible to determine the exact position of the ostium, allowing proper stent positioning (Fig 4.2)
- place a second guidewire, preferably with a distal loop, on the circumflex branch to implant the ostial stent with a jailed wire on the LCX as the distal point of reference; the guidewire is then withdrawn at a later phase (Fig 4.3)
- *tail wire or Szabo technique* [124, 125]: this technique uses a second angioplasty guidewire positioned in the aorta to anchor the stent at the ostial location by passing the proximal end of the anchor wire through the last cell of the stent. The stent travels over both the primary wire into the artery and the anchor wire, which stops the forward motion of the stent at the aorto-ostial junction. This technique prevents the stent, once placed, from sliding into the LMCA, due to the cardiac cycle, allowing proper ostium coverage (Fig 4.4).

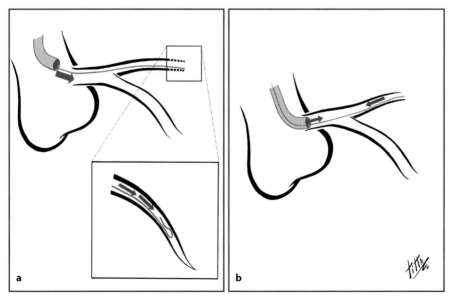

Fig. 4.2 Left main coronary artery engagement. **a** Deployment of coronary wire with loop distal to the vessel's periphery. **b** Withdrawing and pushing the guidewire leads to guiding catheter advance and recoil, respectively

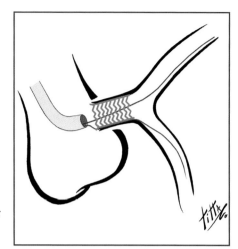

Fig. 4.3 The coronary guidewire with distal loop is placed at the LCX periphery and jailed during stent deployment. It is useful for a very short LMCA ostial stenosis with probable bifurcation involvement

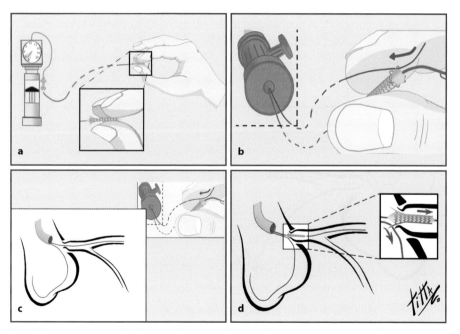

Fig. 4.4 Stent tail wire or Szabo technique. **a, b** Before wiring the stent in the guiding catheter, a coronary anchor wire is deployed through the distal strut. **c** The stent is advanced in the catheter along the first guidewire up to the vessel's origin together with the anchor wire, which is left outside the coronary vessel ostium in the aorta. The stent is deployed in the coronary artery vessel up to the ostial lesion; the anchor wire blocks it from further advancing beyond the ostium. **d** The stent is released at low pressure and expanded at high pressure after removing the anchor wire

This technique is seldom used in practice owing to its greater complexity and because simpler and more rapid alternatives are available

- *placement of a second guidewire in the aorta* (Fig 4.5): a second guidewire is passed through the guiding catheter and then released in the aorta tracing its outline, preventing selective cannulation of the ostium by the guiding catheter, in order to precisely determine the LMCA origin
- two new devices have recently been produced to minimize the potential pitfalls linked to LMCA ostial treatment: Ostial Pro [134] and Square One [135]. The former is a nitinol-based, four-distal-arm device, utilized in conjunction with standard stenting techniques to assist in accurately placing stents. After deploying the coronary guidewire in the vessel's periphery and stent passing the ostial lesion, the nitinol device's self-expanding part, once it has reached the guiding catheter's exit port, opens into four arms, which prevent selective catheter engagement, hence tracing the profile of the aorta and coronary artery ostium, and positioning the coronary guidewire coaxially to the vessel for accurate stent placement [134]. The latter is a stent that is pre-mounted over a balloon with a separate proximal flare region, expanded by a large balloon, providing both tactile and visual localization of the ostium. The cylindrical portion of the stent is then expanded. This system ensures accurate stent positioning at the ostium and its complete coverage, as well as easy vessel recannulation [135].

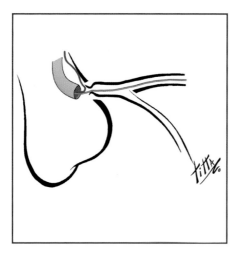

Fig. 4.5 A second guidewire opening into the aorta prevents selective engagement of the guiding catheter in the coronary artery ostium

4.3.1
Pitfalls

During LMCA ostial stenting some complications, which can be effectively resolved, may occur. These are described under the headings that follow.

4.3.1.1
Elastic Recoil

This is the most frequent occurrence and is the result of the elasticity of the ostium described above and of its anatomical characteristics (take-off) (Fig. 4.6). The possible solutions are:
- overstretching with a non-compliant balloon with a large diameter; the solution is not very effective and can easily lead to ostial damage of the vessel during the periprocedural phase (dissection) and/or in the follow-up (restenosis and/or recoil) (Fig. 4.7)
- "sandwich" stenting, which consists of implanting a second stent inside the first (Figs. 4.8, 4.9).

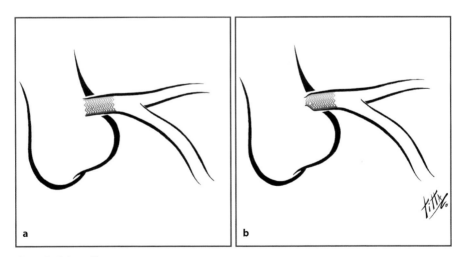

Fig 4.6 Ostial recoil

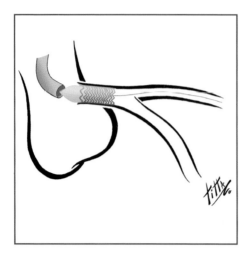

Fig 4.7 Post-dilatation, at high pressure, of the ostial stent with a non-compliant balloon

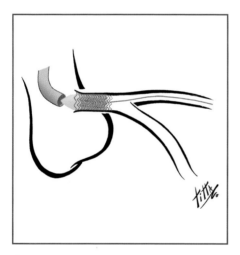

Fig. 4.8 "Sandwich stenting": implantation of another stent inside the former, slightly prolapsing into the aorta to allow "flaring"

In most cases, ostial recoil can be easily solved without further complications. Out of 119 patients with ostial disease treated at our institution, during the procedure it occurred in only nine patients (7.6%). Just one case required elective surgery because of unsolved recoil after a sandwich technique; in all the other cases another stent was implanted to solve the problem. Currently the

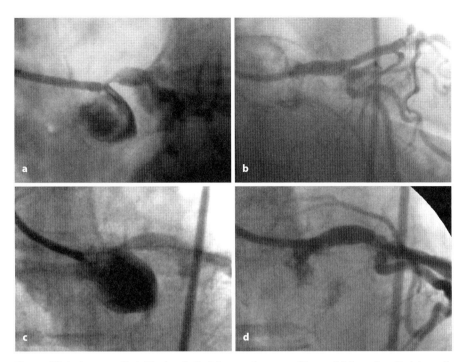

Fig. 4.9 Clinical case. **a** Ostial lesion. **b** Ostial stent placement (Taxus 4.0/8 mm). **c** Ostial recoil. **d** Deployment of a second stent (Taxus 4.0/8 mm) (sandwich stenting)

clinical follow-up of these patients is 46 ± 12 months. An 86-year-old patient with low systolic function indices (LVEF 25%) died as a result of ingravescent heart failure 14 months following the procedure; at angiographic follow-up two patients showed hemodynamically significant restenosis.

4.3.1.2
Stent Hang-out

If the ostial stent protrudes by a few millimeters into the aorta, it does not affect patency or stent function nor does it give rise to any mechanical impediment for the aortic valve; but it may become a problem in cases of a new coronary angiography or angioplasty (Fig. 4.10). In these cases, utmost attention is required during recannulation of the stent protruding into the aorta, to avoid damaging the latter. After accurate selection of the most appropriate catheter, it is possible to:

- use a 0.35" guidewire to alter the curve and orientation of the distal part of the catheter, making it more appropriate for cannulation

- insert the coronary guidewire during semi-selective cannulation. Once the guidewire is placed at the vessel's edge, the catheter can be oriented to allow coaxial positioning compared to the stent. In this case the main difficulty lies in inserting the coronary guidewire and placing it at the edge of the vessel without adequate support (Fig. 4.11). The support of the guidewire can also be

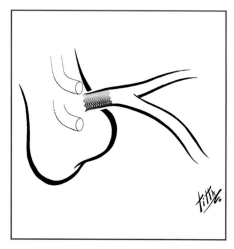

Fig. 4.10 Stent hang-out

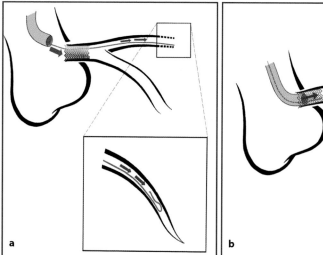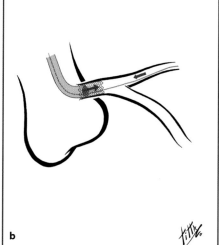

Fig. 4.11 Stent hang-out: first-choice solution to cannulate. **a** Semi-selective cannulation of the coronary artery and placement with distal loop of the coronary guidewire with intermediate support. **b** Withdrawing the guidewire leads to guiding the catheter advance along the coronary guidewire with subsequent selective cannulation of the guiding catheter into the hanging-out stent

augmented by inserting a deflated balloon catheter until it reaches the coronary artery.

If it is not possible to easily and quickly cannulate the vessel in an emergency situation, the guidewire can be inserted into a lateral stent cell and the struts can be crushed to create a neo-ostium (Fig. 4.12).

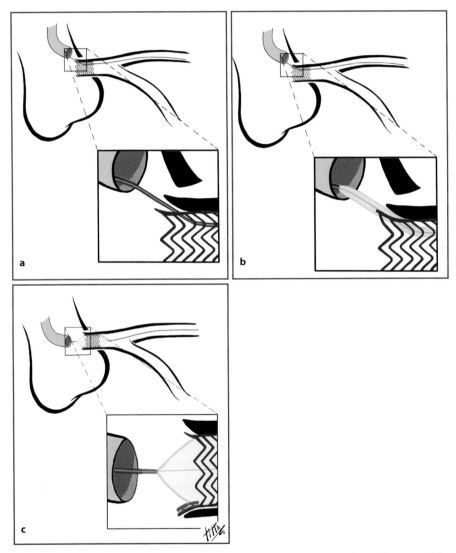

Fig. 4.12 Stent hang-out: second-choice solution to cannulate. **a** In emergencies, side access of the stent opening in the aorta is possible. **b**, **c** Subsequent crush, with a balloon, of the stent's lateral strut

4.3.1.3
Ostial Missing

In cases of guiding catheter instability, lesion pre-dilatation may complicate proper stent placement, further favoring the movement transmitted during systole and diastole from the guiding catheter to the delivery catheter. In these cases, stent entrapment in the lesion is useful, as it increases stability and reduces movement during implantation.

In cases of anterograde stent shift during implantation, another stent needs to be placed for proper ostium coverage (Fig. 4.13). Another occurrence, albeit rare, is balloon entrapment in the stent's struts following implantation. It may happen that the balloon drags the stent along with it into the aorta during post-stenting withdrawal. Usually this occurs with stents, and hence balloons, of larger size, but nevertheless underestimated compared to vessel diameter. In such cases an attempt needs to be made to re-inflate the balloon in the aorta, in order to entrap the stent and then withdraw the entire system composed of the guiding catheter, coronary guidewire, balloon, and stent back to the sheath. If the patient shows signs of clinical instability, it is highly recommended that these maneuvers be put off until the plaque is stabilized by implanting another stent, passing it through the one opening into the aorta (Figs. 4.14, 4.15).

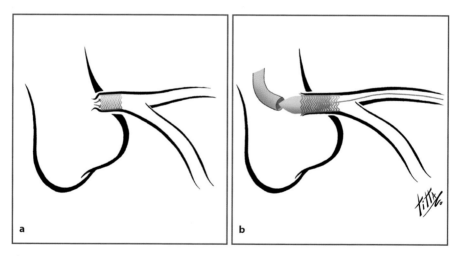

Fig. 4.13 Ostial missing. **a, b** Sandwich stenting, deployment of a second stent, inside the former, in a lesion left exposed following anterograde shift of the first stent

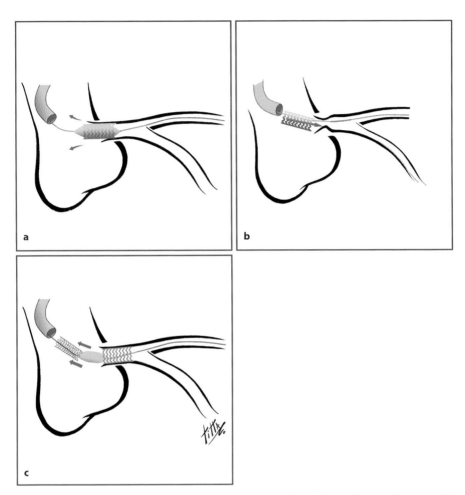

Fig. 4.14 Proximal stent sliding. **a** After expanding the stent, the balloon adheres to the stent with displacement towards the aorta. **b** Deployment of the second stent with ostial lesion stabilization. **c** Recovery of the displaced stent opening in the aorta

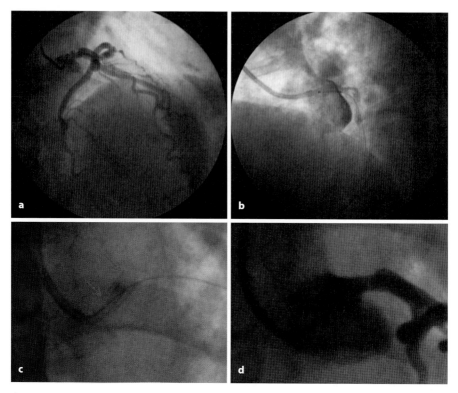

Fig. 4.15 Proximal stent sliding: clinical case. **a** Ostial lesion (probable dissection due to catheter).
b Placement of ostial stent underestimated compared to vessel diameter (Taxus 3.5/8 mm).
c Displaced stent in aorta (*arrows*). **d** Placement of a second stent (Driver 4.0/9 mm) inside the
first one

4.3.1.4
Sliding

See body lesions (Section 4.4).

4.3.1.5
Proximal–Distal Dissection

Retrograde dissection of the ostium towards the aorta is a rather rare event.
When the extent of this dissection is minor, serial control with transesophageal
echocardiography (TEE) and CT angiography is highly recommended. In this
case, considering that it is minor dissection in the direction of the blood flow,
keeping the pressure values low will suffice. When a progression of the lesion is

observed, a cardiac surgery consultation needs to be requested. Covered stents occluding the entry port can also be used in these cases. However, this solution is seldom used owing to the high frequency of restenosis, which greatly limits the use of this type of stent except in emergency situations.

Anterograde dissection affecting the body and/or bifurcation is treated by stenting. Dissection at the distal edge of the stent implanted on the LMCA ostium often occurs because the extent of the disease has been underestimated. Partial plaque coverage is often the cause of dissection (geographical missing).

4.4
Body Lesions

The technical approach adopted for LMCA body lesions (body or shaft) is usually the simplest. The result of the procedure and the medium- and long-term outcome are excellent as well. However, in this subset of lesions too, there can be potential pitfalls requiring, at times, recourse to particular expedients. Many are similar to those already described for ostial lesions. Nonetheless, some considerations need to be made.

4.4.1
Elastic Recoil

This is very rare; when it occurs, the same treatment described for ostial lesions is to be adopted.

4.4.2
Difficult Stent Centering

The distal edge is often located very close to the bifurcation and in case of oscillation, as for the ostium, it is preferable not to pre-dilate the lesion, so that the stent remains entrapped, allowing proper placement.

4.4.3
Sliding

Stent sliding can be immediate or late. It usually depends on the mismatch between stent diameter and LMCA diameter. The situations that may occur and their possible solutions are:

- *the stent slides uncovering the stenosis*: in this case a stent with a larger size is to be placed. If the first stent has already reached its maximum diameter, the purpose of the additional stent is to entrap the former, engaging it, and, at the same time, to cover the lesion left exposed. If sliding is due instead to inadequate dilatation, the implantation of an additional stent also serves to adequately dilate the former. In case of entrapment, the entire segment covered by the stent is to be homogeneously expanded in order to prevent distortion of the struts owing to size mismatch
- *the stent cannot be further expanded and it undergoes anterograde shift*: as a rule, during its shift, it fails to pass the bifurcation. When using BMS, dead room between the stent and vessel wall does not cause thrombosis, as the stent is completely covered with neo-intima in the course of time without further exposure to the risk of thrombosis (Fig. 4.16)

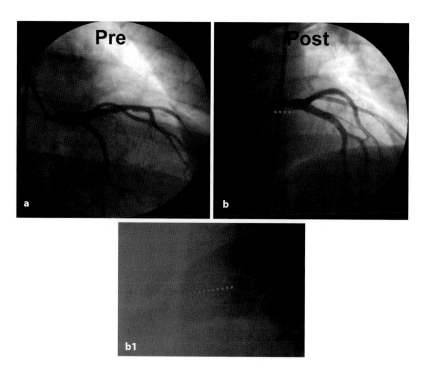

Fig. 4.16 Distal stent sliding: clinical case. **a** Basal. **b** After stent placement [Technic 3.5/12 mm – see radiopaque markers at the edge of the stent (*dotted lines*)]. (*cont.* ➤)

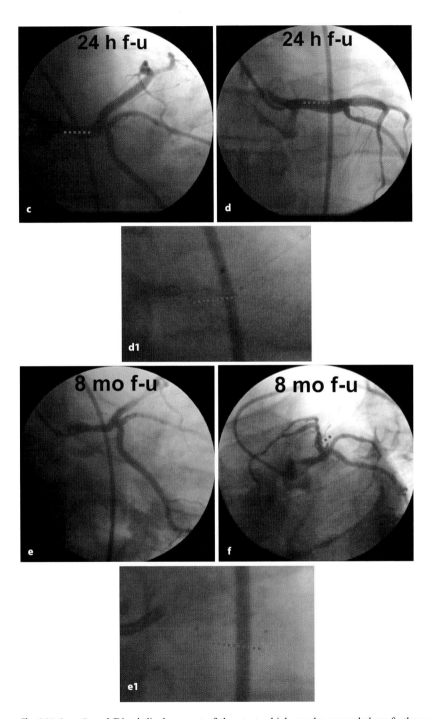

Fig. 4.16 (*cont.*) **c, d** Distal displacement of the stent which can be expanded no further. **e, f** At 8-month angiographic follow-up, the stent has slid further forward at the bifurcation

- *the stent is displaced reaching the bifurcation and remains open at the origin of the main branches*: one possible solution is to withdraw the stent, trying to entrap it after inflating a balloon inside it, or an attempt can be made to stabilize its position with a kissing balloon (Figs. 4.17, 4.18), or the distal edge of the stent can simply be flared to get stable positioning at the ostium of the LCX and/or LAD. A second proximal stent is hence implanted, to cover the lesion that is left uncovered.

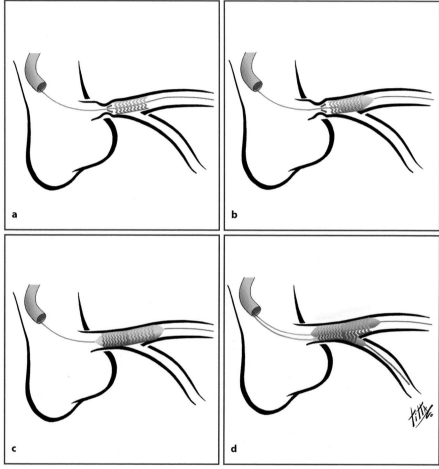

Fig. 4.17 Distal stent sliding. **a** The first stent is displaced and engaged at the origin of a bifurcation branch. **b** Balloon stabilization. **c** Deployment of a second stent of a larger size covering the lesion and jailing the former stent, hence avoiding further movements. **d** The kissing balloon procedure is completed

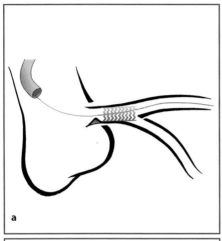

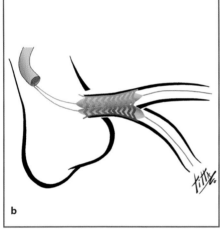

Fig. 4.18 Distal stent sliding. **a** Sliding of the stent up to the bifurcation. **b** Placement of another stent on the lesion left exposed, and stabilization of the stents at the bifurcation with the kissing balloon technique by making the two balloons hang out a few millimeters into the bifurcation branches

4.4.4
Proximal–Distal Dissection

Proximal and distal dissection following stenting of the LMCA body is usually the consequence of underestimating the lesion, which is treated with a stent that is shorter than needed. This requires treatment of the proximal and distal part of the lesion as described below. However, if the main branch is very long, dissection can be effectively sealed with further stenting (Fig. 4.19).

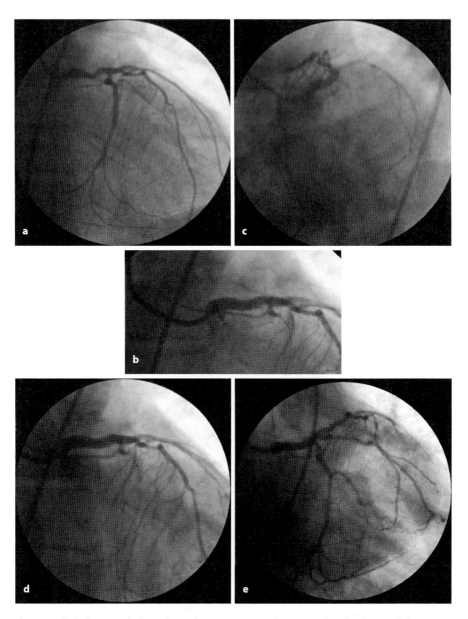

Fig. 4.19 Clinical case of dissection after LMCA stenting. **a** Lesion in the medial LMCA. **b, c** Dissection at the distal edge after stent deployment due to geographical missing (Taxus 3.5/ 12 mm), with acute LCX occlusion. **d** Placement of another stent on the distal edge (Taxus 3.5/8 mm, use of 2b/3a glycoprotein inhibitors). **e** Angiographic follow-up at 8 months, patent LCX

4.5
Distal Lesions

This is definitely the most challenging subset of lesions when dealing with the LMCA. Surgery is often considered in this set of lesions, especially when other main vessel disease co-exists. Before treating this lesion, several aspects need to be considered and these include bi-/trifurcation anatomy, plaque layout and composition, and the patient's clinical status. Many definitions have been suggested for a coronary bifurcation lesion. A recent consensus document [136] by the European Bifurcation Club defines a coronary bifurcation lesion as "any lesion adjacent to or involving a significant side branch". "Significant" is understood as any side branch deemed important by the operator, considering the patient's overall clinical picture. Many classifications published in recent years have assessed, above all, the distribution of the atherosclerotic plaque, but they require a huge mnemonic effort, which hence greatly limits their application. The recent Medina classification [137], while consisting of a summation of prior classifications from which it takes all the characteristics, is very concise and does not require great efforts to memorize it. It divides the bifurcation into three segments [main branch (MB), proximal, distal, and side branch (SB)] (Fig 4.20), and assesses whether or not there is disease causing stenosis >50%

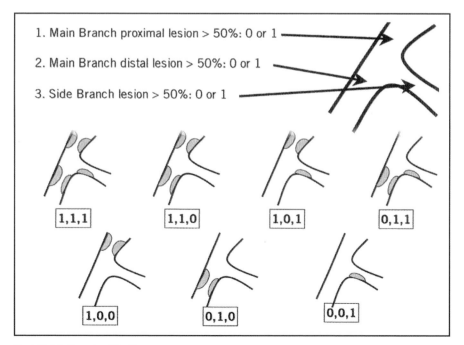

Fig. 4.20 Medina classification

of vessel diameter in each segment, assigning a value of 1 or 0, respectively. Therefore, three simple numbers make it possible to identify the plaque distribution pattern in the bifurcation.

Lesions affecting the distal LMCA should always be considered as bifurcation (or trifurcation) lesions. However, the Medina classification, which fits other types of coronary artery bifurcation well, does not provide important or essential details for distal LMCA percutaneous treatment. In this case, besides the distribution of atherosclerotic plaque, it is essential to assess the anatomy of the distal LMCA, a key factor in the choice of the percutaneous technique to be adopted: single- or two-stent.

For instance, a retroflex LCX originating from the LMCA and forming an acute angle (Fig. 4.21) requires different and often much more complex strategies compared to a LCX with right or obtuse angle. In this case, placing a second stent in the SB requires maneuvers to increase support and hence the possibility of pushing the stent (anchor balloon technique, buddy wires, etc); in addition, the stent will be exposed to repeated mechanical stress in the course of time due to the vessel's retroflex anatomy. It accounts for the generation of a turbulent blood flow and an increased risk of ISR at angiographic follow-up. When dealing with a trifurcation, besides the bifurcation angle, the relevance of

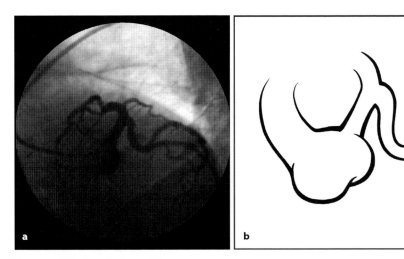

Fig. 4.21 LCX with retroflex origin

the third branch, the angles, and the distances between the origins of the vessels needs to be assessed (Figs. 4.22, 4.23). The LMCA size and the difference in size compared to its branches are to be taken into account as well (Fig. 4.24). An extremely proximal origin of any other collateral vessels of the LAD or LCX (Fig. 4.25), distal angles of the LMCA, and angles of the LAD (Fig 4.26) determine different therapeutic approaches.

As regards lesion distribution, it must be considered that, unlike other coronary artery bifurcations, LMCA bifurcation usually has a much broader carina. Therefore, there can be a larger number of lesion patterns compared to a bifurcation located in another coronary artery segment (Fig. 4.27).

The number of possible distributions of plaque over the LMCA bifurcation increases in cases of trifurcation and they can occur in various anatomical scenarios.

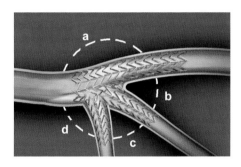

Fig. 4.22 Schematic overview of trifurcation stenting for the various measurements and angles (*a, b, c, d*) (adapted Medina classification)

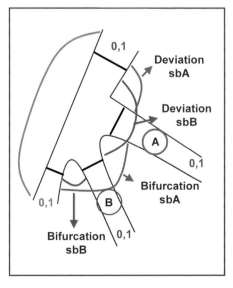

Fig. 4.23 Detailed schematic overview of trifurcation stenting for the various measurements and angles (adapted Medina classification)

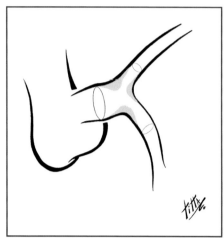

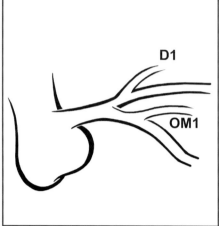

Fig 4.24 Size discrepancy between the LMCA and its bifurcation branches, LAD and LCX

Fig. 4.25 Early origin of an obtuse marginal branch (*OM1*) and diagonal branch (*D1*)

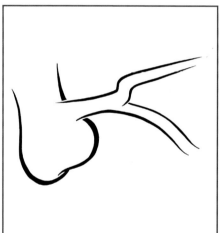

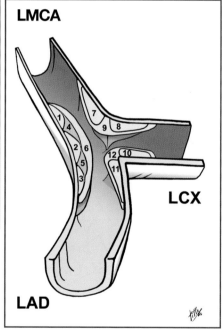

Fig. 4.26 Angulated LAD course after take-off

Fig. 4.27 Plaque distribution in bifurcation

For all these reasons, it is impossible to codify the best strategy for all types of diseased LMCA. However, it is possible to chart out a standardized map of the main problems with the relevant technical solutions. Standardizing data from different patient populations and extrapolating results that are passed off as universal should also be shunned.

It can be easily and rather simplistically stated that the proper application of any technique whatsoever is essential to obtain the immediate result. By contrast, every technique seems to have different results at follow-up.

LMCA lesion patterns also include those cases with isolated lesion of the LAD and LCX ostia (Fig. 4.28). Ostial lesions (<2 mm from take-off) anatomically belong to the LAD and LCX, respectively, even though their treatment inevitably involves the distal LMCA. This happens for various reasons, one or more of which always presents in the set of LAD/LCX ostial PCIs: plaque shift, proximal trauma in the case of stenting, kissing balloon, protection of the distal LMCA with a balloon inflated from the LMCA to the non-diseased branch, geographical missing with incomplete plaque coverage or excessive stent protrusion into the LMCA bifurcation, or ostial elastic recoil with a need for larger balloons.

The obvious consequences are: first, ostial LAD and LCX lesions need a careful follow-up monitoring, similar to distal LMCA lesions; and second, these lesions should be "ab initio" treated as distal LMCA disease.

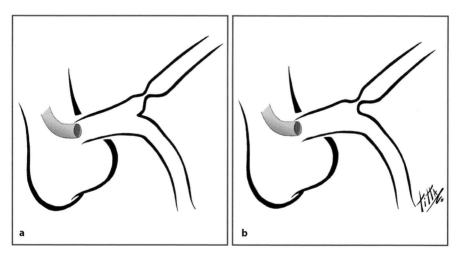

Fig. 4.28 Ostial lesion. **a** Isolated LAD ostial lesion: <2 mm from the bifurcation carina; **b** >2 mm from the bifurcation carina

4.5.1
Guiding Catheter

If the choice of the guiding catheter is of relative importance for the ostium and LMCA body, it becomes essential for treating a bifurcation. The guiding catheter must ensure:

- *back-up*: Amplatz or XB catheters are guiding catheters that generally afford optimal support in order to rapidly achieve success in a complex case of LMCA PCI. In a long and tortuous aorta it is recommended to use a long, metal reinforced, sheath. This ensures greater guiding catheter stability, overcoming any irregularities in the course and the drift of any twists and stenoses, especially in the presence of kinking and/or ileofemoral stenoses
- *coaxial orientation*: the choice of the appropriate curve depends on the dimensions (width and length) of the ascending aorta and aortic arch. Therefore, every individual case should be carefully assessed by the operator in order to choose the most appropriate measure. Often, in cases of difficult stent crossing, with calcified plaques or a sharp angle at the LCX or LAD origin, it is enough to change the entry angle of the guiding catheter in the coronary artery (pulling it back and/or rotating it) to achieve co-axial placement and favor stent passage. The same may occur during the passage of the balloon used for the final kissing balloon
- *diameter*: when treating a LMCA bifurcation lesion, a 7 or 8 Fr catheter is needed in order to favor the use and exchange of devices as well as their simultaneous use, as in the case of a kissing balloon or kissing stents. An 8 Fr catheter is recommended when a triple kissing balloon is envisaged, treating a trifurcation lesion, when a rotablator with a burr over 1.75 mm is used, or in emergent procedure conditions.

4.5.2
PCI Wires

As a rule of thumb, each commonly used guidewire (Table 4.1) can be used for distal LMCA PCI. In general, spring soft-tipped guidewires with or without hydrophilic coating (BMW or BMW Universal) are a safe and reliable choice. However, in the case of a complex lesion, winding SBs, or the presence of a diseased SB, it is recommended to use soft plastic guidewires ensuring better traceability (Pilot series, Choice, etc). In order to perform re-crossing on the SB, plastic-type guidewires with a high support capacity are recommended. If necessary (e.g. very acute bifurcation angles, and tight, eccentric stenoses, complicating the deployment of the various devices, balloons, and stents), guidewires providing high support (BHW, Grand Slam, Choice Extra Support) are useful.

Let us now analyze the various techniques for distal LMCA stenting.

4.6
Percutaneous Coronary Intervention Technique

The choice of strategy depends on several factors, some of which are self-evident but seldom admitted:

- *operator experience*: many operators prefer some treatment techniques compared to others, owing to a greater confidence gained with experience
- *operator timing*: some operators choose to adopt one technique instead of another as they prefer techniques requiring less time. A shorter procedure time also entails a lower risk of complications such as periprocedural acute thrombosis
- *number of operators*: if there are two or more operators, they may prefer a more complex technique, nonetheless assuring a better immediate result
- *the patient's clinical presentation*: in the case of acute coronary syndrome, it is preferable, when possible, to use the least number of stents, in order to reduce possible hemodynamic destabilization. In this context, the number of implanted stents and the length of the treated lesion segment are correlated with a higher risk of acute and subacute stent thrombosis [138–143]. Therefore, a technique aimed at stabilizing the plaque in the least possible time is useful and necessary, even at the cost of a fairly good yet not optimal angiographic result. In this case, the procedure can be revised or improved at a later time, once the patient has been stabilized
- *lesion characteristics and distribution*: basic principles for choosing a single versus two-stent procedure
- *importance of the vessels to be treated* (presence of necrosis, right or left prevalence, vessel size, etc): in order to reduce procedural risk, treatment should be limited only to vessels supplying viable myocardial tissue. The treatment of lesions in vessels with a small diameter is avoided, as these make a minor contribution to overall myocardial vascularization while increasing procedural risk and cardiac adverse events at follow-up. In the case of multi-vessel disease, a staged approach for revascularization is preferable. Procedural risk should be assessed depending on the presence of a minor right coronary artery (RCA) and hence a left prevalence or the presence of a diseased dominant artery for the right territory
- *field of scientific interest*: use of newly introduced techniques or devices.

4.6.1
Lesion Preparation

The treatment of distal LMCA lesions, owing to the clinical relevance of the vessels originating from it, requires protection of the two bifurcation branches by wiring. Moreover, regardless of the technique chosen for a lesion affecting the whole bifurcation, kissing balloon pre-stenting is always recommended to duly prepare the lesion for the subsequent placement of stents. Generally speaking, the preference is for semi-compliant balloons, but caution is needed to avoid overestimating the diameter of the balloon selected to dilate the SB in order to avoid iatrogenic lesions in the proximal third of the SB. In the case of highly calcified lesions, IVUS is useful in selecting the use of non-compliant balloons and/or debulking techniques (see Chapter 3).

4.6.2
Single Stent Technique

Undoubtedly, this is the simplest approach. It comprises various techniques all sharing the same purpose: "one stent implantation as intention to treat". It is, of course, recommended in cases in which the lesion is limited to one or two segments of the bifurcation.

4.6.2.1
T-provisional

The most commonly used single technique is the T-provisional, understood as stenting of the main vessel across the SB (Fig. 4.29) [144]. In the distal LMCA, in the vast majority of cases, stent implantation with this technique is performed to the benefit of the LAD, for several reasons:
- the LAD commonly has a slightly smaller size compared to the distal LMCA, thus allowing the use of a single stent to cover both the LMCA lesion and the lesion in the ostial–proximal LAD segment
- if the feeding myocardial tissue is preserved, when the LAD is functionally more important for the patient than the LCX (LCX of small size)
- in general, the angle between the distal LMCA and the LCX origin makes stent implantation in the LCX rather cumbersome, as LCX ostium is more prone to develop ISR compared to the LAD

However, some situations may warrant stenting for the LCX, among which are:

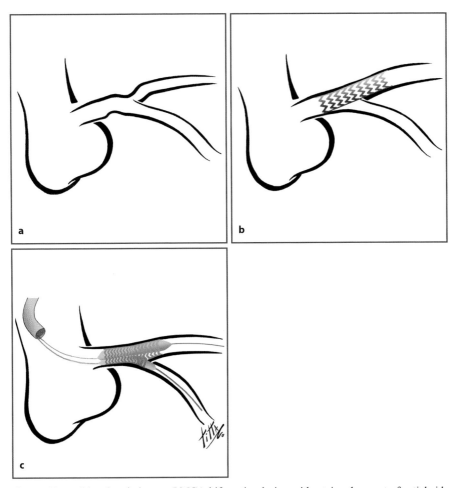

Fig. 4.29 T-provisional technique. **a** LMCA bifurcation lesion without involvement of ostial side branch. **b** Stent positioning LMCA-LAD across LCX. **c** Final kissing balloon

- treatment of protected LMCA with occluded LAD revascularized by functioning by-pass or in the presence of heterocoronary collaterals (from the RCA)
- treatment of unprotected LMCA in the presence of occluded LAD, but with homocoronary collaterals (from the LCX)
- absence of LAD functional importance (patients with prior acute myocardial infarction in the area feeding the LAD, without residual viability)
- distribution of the atherosclerotic disease mainly in the ostium of the LCX and distal LMCA without LAD involvement, in the presence of an angle allowing LCX stenting
- an unfavorable angle between the distal LMCA and LAD.

4.6.2.2
Skirt

This is a technique to treat distal LMCA when the disease does not affect the ostia of the daughter branches, in the presence of an acute bifurcation angle (Fig. 4.30). It consists of implanting a single stent near the bifurcation carina without the involvement of the LAD and LCX ostia. After re-crossing of the SBs, the procedure is completed with a final kissing balloon. Due attention must be paid to choosing the sizes of the balloons, which must hang out by no more than a few millimeters in the ostium of the two branches. A final kissing

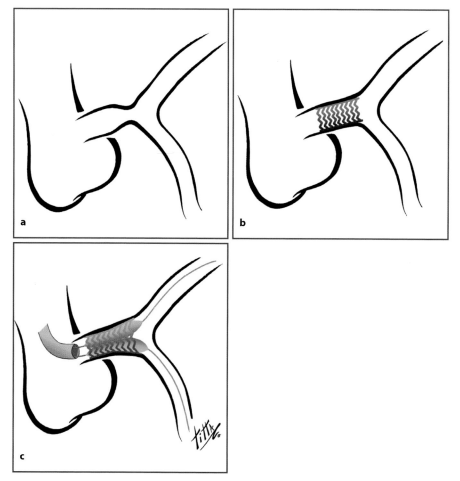

Fig. 4.30 Skirt technique. **a** Lesion of LMCA bifurcation. **b** Implantation of stent at the site of bifurcation. **c** Final kissing balloon

balloon is not necessary if no distress is observed in the ostium of either the LAD or the LCX, due to the presence of some stent strut hang-out (IVUS can be applied in this case) [145, 146]. Recently, conceptual developments of this technique have led to the creation of a dedicated system for bifurcation treatment that is now commercially available: the Devax system (Fig. 4.31) [147]. In the case of onset of dissection in the LAD/LCX ostia, or plaque shift determining significant stenoses, this procedure can be completed with the implantation of one or two stents in the daughter branches.

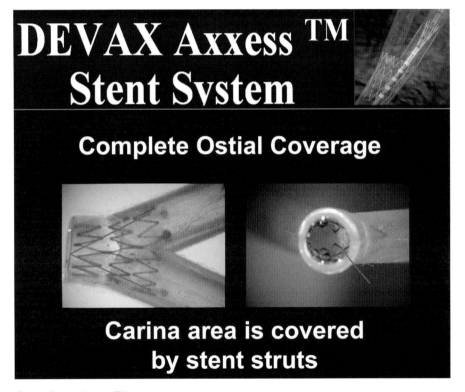

Fig.4.31 Devax Axxess™ stent system

4.6.2.3
Isolated Treatment of LAD and LCX Ostia

As mentioned previously, in many cases the plaque may be selectively located
in the LAD or LCX ostium (Fig. 4.32). If the distance between the plaque and
the bifurcation carina is <2 mm, these lesions are considered as affecting the
distal LMCA. In these cases, in our opinion, this lesion should be treated by
reconstructing part of the carina. Nonetheless, many operators prefer isolated
treatment of the ostium of the affected branch [148]. Besides technical problems

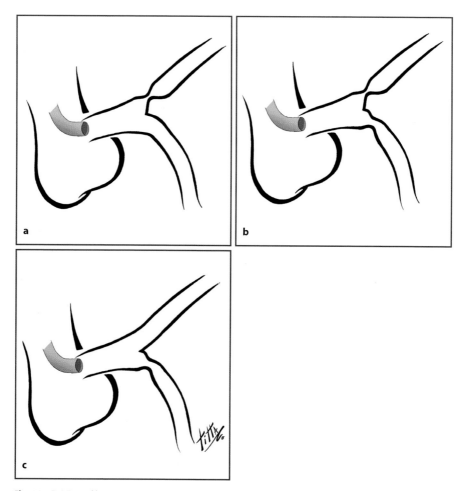

Fig. 4.32 LAD and/or LCX ostial disease. **a** Isolated LAD ostial disease. **b** LAD and LCX ostial
disease. **c** Isolated LCX disease

linked to the disease's location, which makes stent placement very cumbersome, the clinical and angiographic outcome of these cases is almost always affected by inevitable trauma to the carina that is not followed by coverage with a stent and/or by retrograde plaque shift in the LMCA or the other coronary artery ostium (Fig. 4.33). However, the likelihood of plaque shift can nonethe-

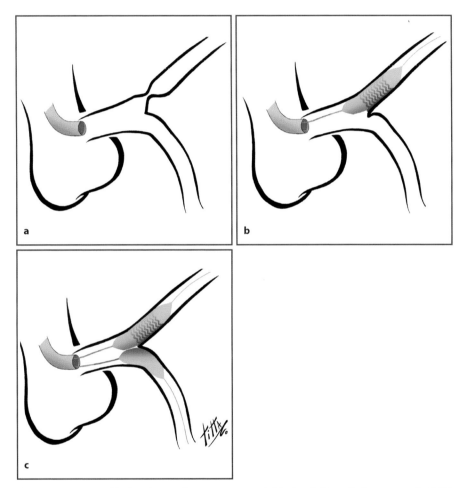

Fig. 4.33 Treatment of isolated LAD disease. **a** LAD ostial lesion. **b** Stent deployment at the LAD ostium with shift of the bifurcation carina and subsequent distress of the LCX ostium. **c** Kissing balloon technique applied in the bifurcation

less be reduced by performing dilatation at low pressure with a semi-compliant balloon in the ostium of the other branch, while implanting the stent. This technique ensures a better immediate result, but it does not guarantee an optimal medium-/long-term result. In our experience, in a retrospective analysis of 77 patients who underwent isolated ostial LAD and/or LCX PCI at our institution from 2002 to 2007, the rate of hierarchical MACE at 21 ± 13 months' follow-up was 25.7%: cardiac death 4.5%, myocardial infarction 1.5%, TLR 16.6%. ST occurred in 6% of cases: definite 1.5%, probable 1.5%, and possible 3.0%. In more detail, it was not possible to ascribe cardiac death to one of the three possible relevant vessels (LAD, LCX, LMCA); conversely, 75% of TLR and 50% of ST occurred in the left main bifurcation (i.e. another location, other than ostial LAD or LCX). It is noteworthy that MACE mainly occurred in patients in whom ostial lesion was treated with one stent placed in the target vessel, hence not covering the LMCA,

4.6.3
Two-stent Technique

Although these approaches are more difficult to perform, they are nonetheless indispensable for widespread disease affecting all three LMCA bifurcation segments (Fig. 4.34). Many authors suggest that, despite the involvement of the SB ostium, coronary artery bifurcations can be treated with a "one-stent technique" if the pathology does not affect more than 3 mm of the SB's proximal section, as the literature has not demonstrated that it affects the clinical outcome in the long run, although the final angiographic result is suboptimal [149]. In our opinion, this view needs to be modified when treating the distal LMCA, owing to the importance of both SBs in the vast majority of cases. Therefore, in case *of in toto* involvement of the bifurcation, a complex approach should always be performed unless the anatomical and clinical conditions when performing double stenting are unfavorable.

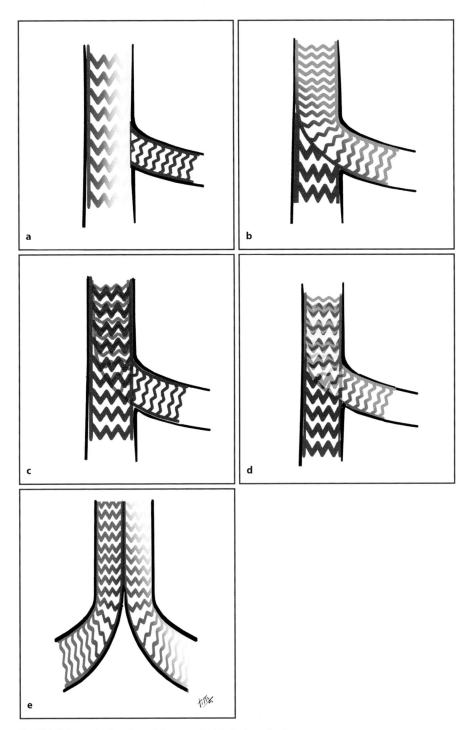

Fig. 4.34 Schematic drawing of the two-stent technique (**a-e**)

4.6.3.1
T-stenting and T-modified Stenting

Standard T-stenting is a technique that can be applied rather well to the LMCA bifurcation. An essential prerequisite is the presence of a bifurcation angle of about 90°; (as in the vast majority of cases) [150]. The steps are very much like those of T-provisional stenting. The only difference is that, from the outset, implantation of a second stent in the SB is planned. This method is complicated by the difficulty in correctly placing the stent at the SB ostium, which may be left exposed, thus giving a suboptimal immediate result and a poor medium-term result, with an increase in the incidence of restenosis, which is usually focal and located at the LCX ostium of (Fig. 4.35). Therefore, the anatomical pattern for its feasibility must be accurately selected. In optimal cases this technique allows a lesser degree of strut overlapping, which, as is well known, is one of the causes of increased restenosis incidence. T-modified stenting is a revised version of this technique, in which the stent is initially implanted in the SB and then in the MB crossing the SB [151].

4.6.3.2
Crush and Mini-crush

Crush stenting was conceived as a solution for difficult T-stenting execution. Incomplete ostium coverage (longitudinal miss) is associated with the presence of residual SB stenoses, which can even be significant, and it is the most likely cause of restenosis. It envisages first the stenting of the SB after positioning the proximal marker a few millimeters (3–4 mm) away from the bifurcation's carina (so that it protrudes considerably in the MB). Then the stent is implanted in the MB, once it has been determined that it is optimally positioned (i.e. that it covers the entire lesion), and the struts of the stent previously implanted in the MB are crushed [152]. Therefore, there are three overlapping layers of struts adhering to the vessel wall in the proximal segment of the bifurcation. The crush technique is marked by an extraordinary immediate result and great ease of performance. However, the results of the first trials have shown a high restenosis rate clearly linked to the extensive presence of "metal" near the origin of the SB. A revised version of this technique is the mini-crush [153], developed to reduce the overlapping of stent struts. This technique is marked by a reduction in the protrusion of the SB stent into the main vessel. The "crush" is performed with a semi-compliant balloon inflated to high pressure before implanting the stent in the MB, in order to adequately crush the stent and improve the expansion of the stent in the MB. The use of this technique has given better results in terms of overall restenosis and isolated restenosis of the SB ostium [153] (Fig. 4.36).

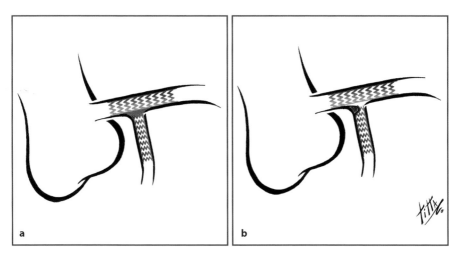

Fig. 4.35 Two-stent technique: ostial LCX missing. **a** Incomplete coverage of LCX ostium. **b** At follow-up, focal restenosis at the LCX ostium

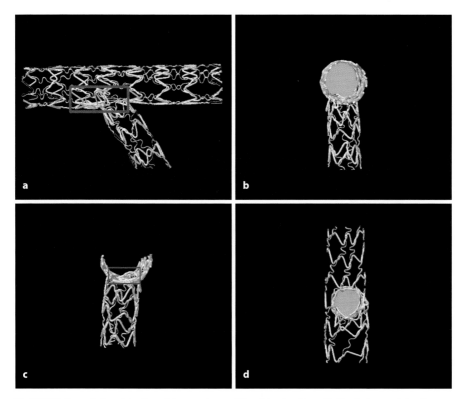

Fig 4.36 Mini-crush (model adapted by courtesy of Ormiston). **a** Longitudinal view, minimal overlapping of struts in the crush site. **b** Cross-section of the stent in the LMCA, regular vessel lumen, symmetric layout of struts. **c** Cross-section of the stent in the LMCA, minimal hang-out of the crushed LCX stent struts in the LMCA. **d** Cross-section of the LCX, ostial stent with symmetrical layout of struts

4.6.3.3
Culotte

Described for the first time by Chevalier et al., this technique it is probably the finest method for the stenting of both branches [154]. The first phase consists of the alternating dilatation of both branches. First, the more angulated branch is stented; then another stent is deployed in the straight branch, through the struts of the former, keeping its proximal part within the stent previously deployed. This method makes it possible to partially cover the proximal segment of the bifurcation with an overlapping of stents (two layers of metal struts adhering to the vessel wall), while each branch is covered by a single stent. In this case, a necessary condition is that the LMCA and the two branches have a similar diameter, because a possible problem is also due to the creation of a third space between the two stents in the proximal main vessel (PMV) (Fig. 4.37), also as a result of tangling of the struts and incomplete expansion of the second stent. This aspect may affect the procedure's result in the long term. Therefore, it is recommended to always post-dilate the PMV with larger-diameter balloons.

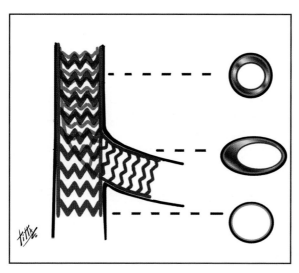

Fig. 4.37 Culotte technique, placement of a stent across the LAD, subsequent placement of a second stent across the former (LMCA-LAD). The schematic drawing shows the cross-section of the LMCA, bifurcation, and LAD

4.6.3.4
"Reverse" techniques

All the aforementioned techniques can also be performed reversely, i.e. by reversing the order of implantation. These changes apply to some specific situations, but they provide the same benefits as the original techniques.

4.6.3.5
V-stenting or V-touching

The use of V-stenting in the diseased distal LMCA is limited to conditions in which the bifurcation angle is <70°; and the disease mainly affects both ostia. The purpose of this technique is not to create a neo-carina and, in order to execute it correctly, the two stents must be deployed simultaneously (Fig. 4.38) [155, 156]. The immediate problems are given by the possible retrograde shift towards the distal LMCA. In this case, two possible solutions are available but neither is optimal: (1) deploy another stent overlapping with one of the two already implanted, crushing the other (excessive overlapping of the struts); or (2) deploy a third stent for the distal section of the LMCA, inevitably leaving the lesion on the carina exposed. At follow-up the effect linked to the trauma in the carina is to be considered. This may greatly impact the incidence of

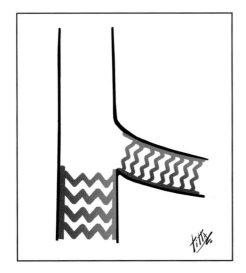

Fig. 4.38 V-stenting technique

restenosis. For these reasons, this technique is used only in very rare cases in which techniques allowing full carina reconstruction cannot be applied, for instance because there is a major difference in diameter between the LMCA and the bifurcation SBs, and hence a single stent cannot be deployed in both the LMCA and the SB.

4.6.3.6
Simultaneous Kissing Stents (SKS)

Despite the simplicity of performance and the good immediate angiographic success it assures, SKS stenting is reserved for a specific anatomical condition: disease affecting the entire bifurcation with a very large LMCA and a major difference in diameter compared to the two SBs. This technique consists in creating a long neo-carina, with a double lumen (double barrel) and double final layer of struts at the center of the main vessel [157, 158] (Figs. 4.39, 4.40). The problems linked to this technique are twisting of the stents following implantation, which often cannot be assessed angiographically and leads in the follow-up to the onset of a peculiar restenosis pattern, called "grotesque". In addition, a double layer at the center of the vessel makes it difficult to plan an appropriate revascularization procedure in the follow-up.

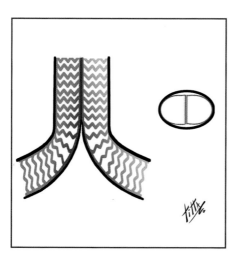

Fig. 4.39 Simultaneous kissing stents (SKS), simultaneous placement of two stents between the LMCA and bifurcation branches. A schematic drawing shows the cross-section of bifurcation

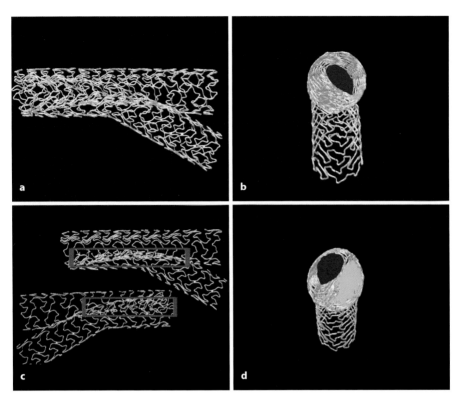

Fig. 4.40 Simultaneous kissing stenting (model adapted by courtesy of Ormiston). **a** Longitudinal view: overlapping of four layers of metal struts on the LMCA, with asymmetric distribution. **b** Cross-section of the stent in the side branch, asymmetric distribution of vessel lumen. **c** Longitudinal view: double lumen in the LMCA upstream of the bifurcation with asymmetrical overlapping of a dual layer of struts. **d** Cross-section of the LMCA: asymmetrical overlapping of metal struts inside the vessel with formation of double lumen

4.7
Treatment Classification

Over the years, alongside the development of PCI, the scientific community has felt the need to create classifications for bifurcation lesion treatment techniques, in order to warrant the most appropriate treatment techniques depending on the type of lesion. Developing a simple yet exhaustive system has proven to be a difficult task for many authors. Among the most widely applied in recent decades, the ICPS (Institut Cardiovasculaire Paris-Sud) classification, issued in 1996 [159] and revised in 2004 following the introduction of new approaches, seems to be difficult to comprehend and memorize today. The European Bifurcation Club has proposed, in its consensus document, a new classification, which, for the first time, introduces simpler visual elements [136]. This classification takes into account initial stent deployment, which often corresponds to a technical strategy related to the importance of the vessel treated first. This classification strives to include all potential technical strategies by describing four ways of beginning the procedure. It is thus divided into four families of treatment corresponding to the suggested acronym "MADS" (Fig. 4.41).

The first family (M for main) starts by stent implantation in the PMV relatively close to the carina. This initial step may be followed by opening of the stent towards both branches (SKIRT technique) [145, 146], with subsequent successive or simultaneous stent placement in one or both distal branches.

The second family (A for Across) starts with the stenting of the PMV to the distal main vessel (DMV) across the SB. This may be the first and the last step of the procedure but may also be followed by the opening of a stent cell with or without kissing balloon inflation towards the SB. After this step, if the delivery of a second stent in the SB is necessary, it is possible to perform T-stenting, TAP (T And small Protrusion) [160], culotte [154], or internal crush configuration [161].

The third family (D for Distal) involves the distal branches and historically starts with simultaneous stent placement at the ostium of both distal branches (V-stenting). A recent variant consists in creating a new carina (the length of which can be determined by QCA) by stent implantation in the proximal segments (SKS). A V-stenting configuration can also be achieved by successive delivery of the stents; a "provisional" variant of SKS consists in delivering a single distal stent by inflating a balloon in the other branch.

The fourth family (S for Side) involves strategies where the SB is stented first, either at ostium level, or with relatively pronounced protrusion into the PMV. The SB stent may be crushed with a balloon inflated in the main vessel (MV), or a second stent may be deployed in the MV across the SB.

This classification applies also for the different dedicated bifurcation stents.

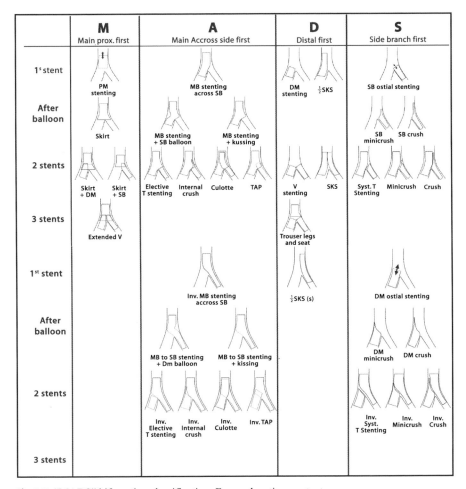

Fig. 4.41 "MADS" bifurcation classification. For explanation see text

For example, the Devax device is deployed by means of a SKIRT technique (M family), while stent delivery systems allowing permanent access to both distal branches are used with the provisional SB stenting strategy of the A family (Frontier Boston, Twinrail Invatec, Nile Minvasys, and so on). An inverted culotte technique is used for deployment of the TRYTON stent and systematic T-stenting for the Cappella stent.

4.7.1
A New Classification for Left Main Coronary Artery Treatment: The "One-Two-Three"

This section aims at sharing our experience in the percutaneous treatment of more than 400 patients with ULMCA lesions at our institution. An analysis of 188 distal LMCA lesions treated has provided food for thought on the development of a classification assessing possible treatment strategies on the basis of the number of stents to be deployed and the technique used. This classification is the "LMCA: one-two-three".

Basically, there are two available techniques: the single-stent technique and the two-stent technique. These should be applied according to plaque distribution and patient clinical conditions (emergent versus others).

Both treatment strategies can be assessed based on the construction of neo-carina (either complete or partial) following stenting. It can hence be concluded that all techniques involving single-stent LMCA treatment (strategy 1) (Fig. 4.42) give a partial formation of neo-carina; by contrast, the most commonly used double-stenting techniques (strategy 2) (Fig. 4.43) assure complete coverage of the bifurcation carina. There are also three seldom used double-stenting techniques, which do not fully cover the carina (strategy 3) (Fig. 4.44).

Based on this conceptual approach, three types of strategies can be identified:
- *strategy 1 – single-stent, incomplete (or partial) neo-carina, defined as type a, b, c, d, e*: strategy 1, if adopted, succeeds in covering the distal LMCA lesion completely in 24% of cases and in about half of these strategy 1a is the most appropriate
- *strategy 2 – two-stent, new carina, defined as type a, b, c, d, e*: strategy 2, if adopted, succeeds in covering the distal LMCA lesion completely in 76% of cases. Although 2a is the most widely used technique, all the other techniques of this group are equally effective in covering the plaque on the bifurcation.
- *strategy 3 – two-stent, incomplete (or partial) neo-carina, type a, b, c*: this is applied only rarely, in situations (<1%) with extremely focalized lesion location.

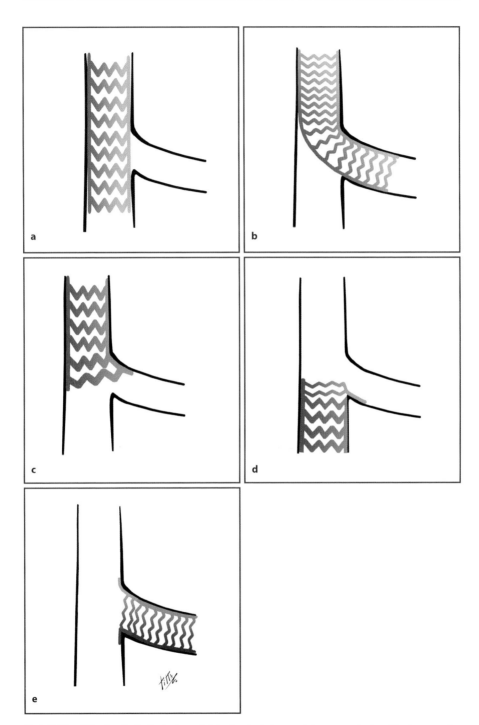

Fig 4.42 Classification 1, 2, 3: strategy 1 (single-stent, incomplete neo-carina). **a** Stent across the LCX. **b** Stent across the LAD. **c** Skirt, stent in the distal LMCA partially covering the bifurcation carina. **d** LAD ostial stent. **e** LCX ostial stent. The part in red is the contact site between the stent and bifurcation chamber

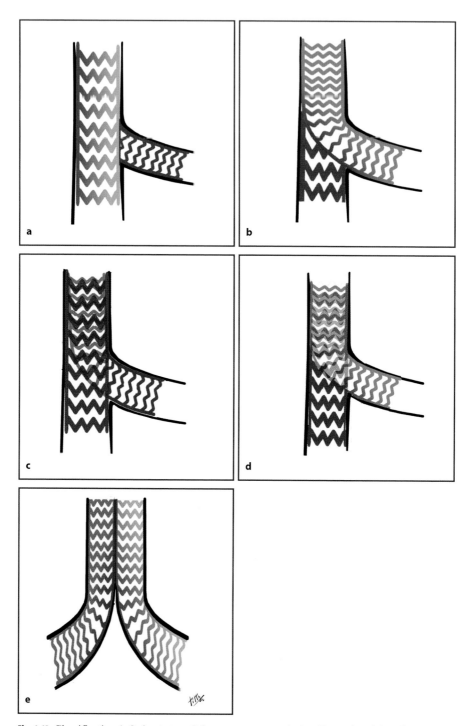

Fig. 4.43 Classification 1, 2, 3: strategy 2 (two-stent, new carina). **a** T, crush, minicrush and vari-ants. **b** Crush, minicrush and variants reverse technique. **c** Culotte. **d** Reverse culotte. **e** Simulta-neous kissing stenting

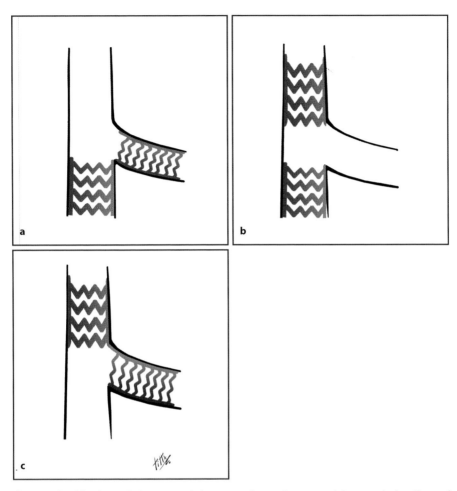

Fig. 4.44 Classification 1, 2, 3: strategy 3 (two-stent, incomplete or partial neo-carina). **a** Stent of both the LAD and LCX ostium. **b** LMCA stenting up to the bifurcation and in ostial LAD without LCX involvement. **c** LMCA stenting up to the bifurcation and in ostial LCX without LAD involvement

Before starting LMCA PCI, it is important to focus attention not only on the immediate procedural result, but also on the follow-up outcome. Successful LMCA treatment in the catheterization lab does not necessarily ensure the best result at follow-up. A proper balance between these two objectives determines the strategy's success.

Therefore, trauma in those vessel segments, in particular the distal section of the bifurcation, which are not expected to be covered by the stent, must be limited.

By way of example, technique 3a, especially indicated for LAD and LCX ostial stenosis, which creates a new partial carina on the distal LMCA, envisages the simultaneous inflation of two balloons in the LMCA, hence potentially causing restenosis on the proximal edge in the follow-up. The same applies, for instance, also for techniques 1c, d, and e: the need to selectively dilate the stent's distal and proximal edge respectively in order to adapt it to bifurcation anatomy inevitably traumatizes the vessel's free walls. In these cases, there are no ad hoc prospective trials corroborating that the two-stent technique (strategy 2), while protecting the vessel's healthy wall, prevents restenosis.

In emergency situations, though, the primary objective is to stabilize the patient as soon as possible. Therefore, a less advantageous technique in the follow-up can prove to be more practical and quicker to apply in the catheterization lab. Technique 2e is of limited elective usefulness and it can be essential in emergency situations in order to stabilize the patient. Unfortunately, in these cases, the problem resurfaces in the follow-up with the onset of ISR.

In this case, restenosis can be treated as follows:
• wire the two stents with two guidewires in parallel and perform re-PCI
• co-axially pass a balloon along the guidewire into the LAD and laterally in the LCX, in order to complete PCI with SB crush (Fig. 4.45).

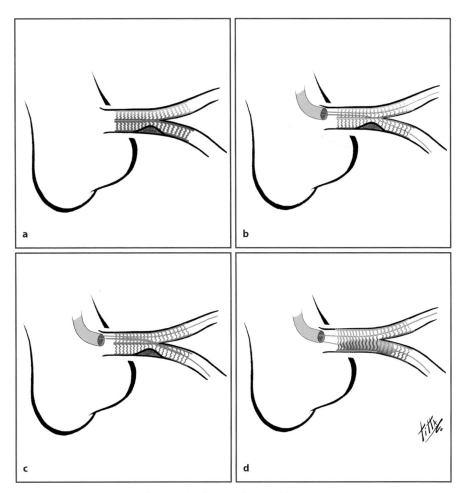

Fig. 4.45 Schematic drawing of restenosis after simultaneous kissing stent employment. **a** Treatment of bifurcation restenosis following SKS technique. **b** Deployment of coronary guidewire to the LAD edge through the LMCA–LAD stent lumen and another guidewire to the LCX edge through the LMCA–LAD stent struts and then the LMCA–LCX stent; **c** Deployment of a coronary balloon across the struts of the two stents. **d** Coronary balloon dilatation with crushing of the central struts of the two stents against the LMCA vessel wall

4.8
Technical Considerations, Pitfalls, Tips, and Tricks

The left main bifurcation is one of the most controversial fields in interventional cardiology because of both the multi-faceted nature of treatment and, especially, the great clinical impact. Our experience has shown that, in order to achieve an optimal procedural result, limiting the risks and ensuring a medium-/long-term positive outcome for the patient, it is extremely important before starting the procedure to carefully assess a series of factors, among which are: (1) bifurcation anatomy; (2) angles between the LMCA and bifurcation branches (LAD, LCX and/or ramus intermedius (RI)); (3) lesion distribution, morphology, and length; (4) the importance of the bifurcation branches; and (5) the patient's clinical status, which also needs to be thoroughly assessed.

It is of note that the "Achilles heel" of the LMCA treatment is the origin of the circumflex branch, which is often the site of restenosis. In this perspective and considering the experience with the population receiving PCI at our institution, we suggest adopting the single-stent technique whenever possible, namely when the disease does not have a major impact on the LCX ostium. This way, not only is it possible to reduce procedure time to the minimum and hence the risk of complications, but also and above all to limit the concentration of metal struts in a site, which, owing to its very anatomical characteristics, is more exposed to continual flow turbulences than others, determining the wavering of the LCX ostium. If it is not possible, double stenting not involving an excessive degree of stent overlapping, like the mini-crush, skirt or V-stenting techniques, is to be preferred. In this case, final kissing balloon inflation is required and non-compliant balloons with sizes no greater than the vessel's reference diameter of the daughter branches should be used. In our experience, marked above all by the use of techniques like T-provisional and mini-crushing, no significant differences have been seen in terms of restenosis incidence among lesions treated with single versus double stenting. Of course, there is still a long way to go, and it is likely that the commercial launch of new dedicated devices will overcome the current limitations.

4.8.1
Crossing Wires

The contemporary use of two or three guidewires during bifurcation treatment requires extremely careful management in order to avoid overlapping, thus making an otherwise simple and rapid procedure potentially risk laden. Crossing would hinder the advance of the various devices through the guiding catheter.

Therefore, in order to distinguish the various guidewires, wet gauzes or color-coded torquers can make work easier and safer. A simple method to avoid crossing a second guidewire with another one at the entrance of the guiding catheter consists of keeping the guide tip in the metallic needle wire introducer during deployment, as long as the simultaneous use of both guidewires is needed. In the case of wire crossing inside the guiding catheter, the only evident sign is the failure of the balloon to advance over the guidewire. In the case of crossing inside the coronary artery, instead, when exerting too much force, besides the catheter failing to advance, there is the risk of recoil of the guiding catheter and hence of the devices and guidewires. This inconvenience can be solved by withdrawing one of the two guidewires, usually the one that is easiest to re-position or the one deployed in the less important vessel, and then to re-deploy it.

4.8.2
Size Discrepancy

According to the fractal law, which applies to bifurcation lesions, the LMCA diameter is always greater than the sum of the two downstream vessels. Therefore, if the intention is to distally cover the LMCA, the following solutions should be applied:

- *the diameter of one of the two vessels is similar to the LMCA's*: deploy the stent from the main to the distal vessel having a similar size (LAD or LCX) and, in the case of the two-stent technique, deploy the second stent in the vessel with the smaller diameter
- *the diameter of both vessels is clearly smaller than that of the LMCA*:
  - (recommended option) use a stent with a high distensibility limit, with an intermediate diameter ranging between the LMCA diameter and the bifurcation diameter and deploy in the LMCA until it sticks out a few millimeters from the daughter branch, releasing it at low pressure. Then, selectively post-dilate the stent segment covering the SB and the segment covering the LMCA, with short non-compliant balloons, each having a diameter duly matching the reference diameter of the two vessels (Figs. 4.46, 4.47). This is essential to avoid the initial stent deployment at nominal pressure values leading to the onset of dissection, plaque shift, or spasm at the distal edge on the SB

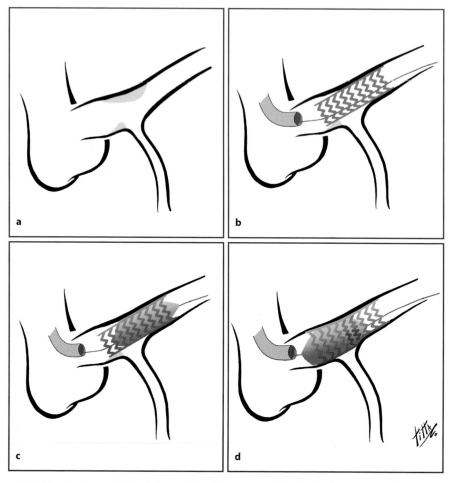

Fig.4.46 Stenting in the LMCA–LAD, size discrepancy. **a** Lesion in the LMCA bifurcation. **b** Provisional stent technique. **c** Dilatation with a balloon that is adequate for the LAD size. **d** Proximal dilatation with a balloon that is adequate for the LMCA size (the procedure is completed with a kissing balloon technique)

– deploy a stent from the LMCA to the juxta-ostial LAD or LCX, and then another stent with or without distal overlap in order to cover the proximal section of the SB; the diameter must match the reference diameter of the SB. In this case post-dilatation of the overlapping point is required with a non-compliant balloon (Fig. 4.48)
– Devax system, see Section 4.6.2.2 (Fig. 4.31).

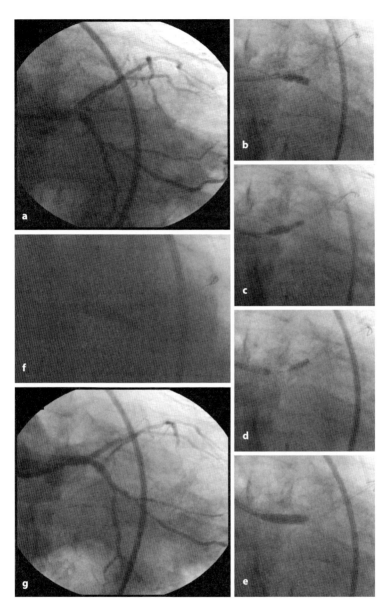

Fig. 4.47 Size discrepancy: clinical case. **a** Critical LMCA bifurcation stenosis. **b** Bifurcation mini-crush technique with stent (Taxus 4.0/8 mm) in ostial LCX. **c** Placement of stent (Taxus 5.0/12) in LMCA–LAD, expanded at low pressure adequate for differentiated stent dilatation. **d** Post-dilatation at high pressure with non-compliant balloon (3.0/8 mm) in ostial LAD. **e** Post-dilatation at high pressure with non-compliant balloon (5.0/10 mm) in the LMCA. **f** Final kissing balloon of bifurcation. **g** Final result

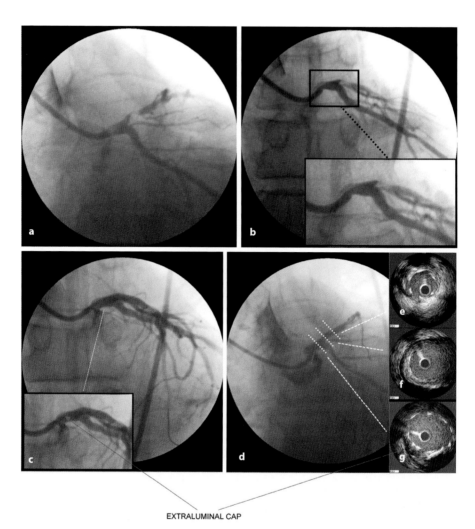

EXTRALUMINAL CAP

Fig. 4.48 Size discrepancy. **a**, **b** LAD–LMCA retrograde helicoid dissection, with size discrepancy between the two vessels. **c** Final result of PCI with implantation of a stent (Cypher 3.0/18 mm) in the ostial LAD and a stent (Taxus 4.0/8 mm) in the LMCA, 1 mm gap between the two stents. **d** Final result of PCI. **e** IVUS imaging of the LAD. **f** IVUS imaging of the distal LMCA, gap between the two stents. **g** IVUS imaging of the LMCA, (*red arrows*: extraluminal cap)

4.8.3
Angulated Take-off

In the case of take-off >90°, various expedients are available to cross the LCX if it requires stenting:

• maneuvering the guiding catheter: deep engagement and rotation, or at the opposite extreme, pulling back and rotating

- buddy wire in the LCX
- using short low-profile and flexible stents (in the case of long lesion using multiple shorter stents from distal-to-proximal)
- anchor technique on the LAD or RI (recommended in the case of failure of the first three solutions above (Fig. 4.49).

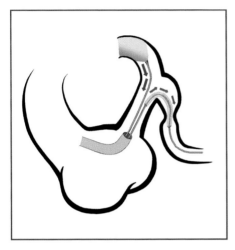

Fig. 4.49 Anchor balloon: anchorage of an inflated balloon on the proximal LAD, hence providing anterior support which facilitates the trackability and successful placement of a balloon (or stent) in the retroflex LCX ostium

4.8.4
Jailed Wire

This technique straightens the vessel reducing the bifurcation angle, identifies the vessel in the case of an eventual abrupt closure after MB stenting, and helps to place the second guidewire correctly for a kissing balloon between the struts and not between the wall and stent. The jailed wire should be withdrawn to avoid the risk of entrapment or tip stretching, once the stent has been expanded only at nominal pressures and once collateral patency has been ascertained.

4.8.5
Buddy Wire

If there is an acute bifurcation angle, excessive vessel winding, or calcification along the vessel's course, crossing a stent might be cumbersome. In this case, parallel deployment of two guidewires helps to increase the support and the anterograde pressure to be exerted in order to cross the obstacle, and moreover decreases the drift between the stent and the vessel wall.

4.8.6
Rotablator

If there is severe calcification liable to potentially limit full stent and balloon expansion, lesion preparation is a priority. The use of a rotablator is beneficial in this case. It can be used in both the LAD and LCX. Considering the dimensions of the LMCA, whose reference diameter is never <3.0 mm, a burr >1.75 mm is always recommended.

This technique is easy to use even in seemingly more severe cases, considering the vicinity of the guiding catheter to the lesion to be treated; it can be easily performed in both daughter vessels of the same patient. The only precaution needed is not to perform rotablation while both guidewires are deployed at the same time (Fig. 4.50).

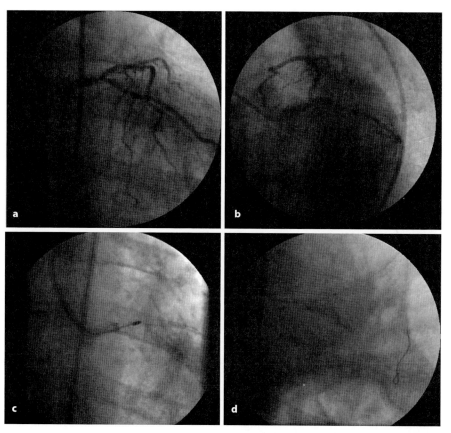

Fig 4.50 Clinical case (fluoroscopic images). **a, b** Calcified lesion of LMCA bifurcation. **c** LMCA–LAD rotablation. **d** T-stenting of bifurcation, placement of stent (Taxus 3.5/12 mm) in the ostial LCX. (*cont.* ⟶)

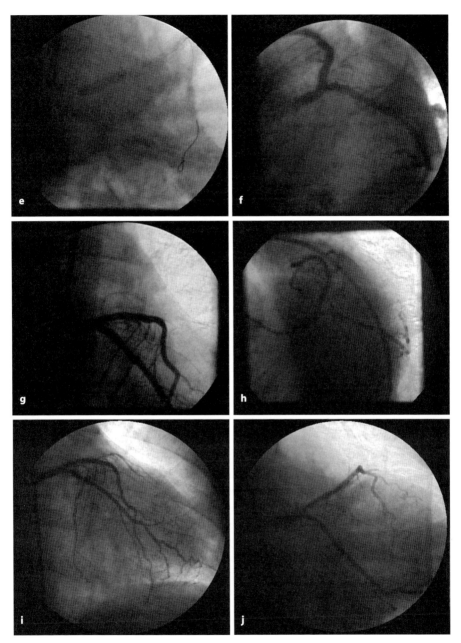

Fig 4.50 (*cont.*) **e** Placement of stent (Taxus 3.5/12 mm) in the LMCA–LAD. **f, g** Final result. **h, i, j** Angiographic follow-up at 24 months, no in-stent restenosis

4.8.7
Cutting Balloons

These are used mainly to treat ISR, especially when it is located in the ostium (LMCA, LAD, LCX); however, at present they are seldom used. Their size often makes insertion through angulated and tight lesions quite cumbersome. Generally speaking, these devices are used in hard calcified lesions, which can be difficult to dilate with compliant or semi-compliant balloons. The use of high-pressure inflation of non-compliant balloons has tremendously limited their use in daily practice and in the LMCA.

4.8.8
Recoil

This mainly occurs at the LMCA ostium (see Section 4.3.1.1). In the distal location it usually occurs in the LCX ostium and, to a lesser degree, in the LAD ostium. It consists of a post-stenting elastic rebound of the vessel at an ostial level, with a narrowing of the vessel's ostial diameter. It is treated with post-dilatation during final kissing balloon application, using non-compliant balloons. It can be prevented in part with the rotablator or cutting balloon. The possible reasons for this event have already been discussed previously.

4.8.9
Thrombus

A thrombus should be resolved, like all those in other sites, with mechanical aspiration, pharmacological therapy, or stenting. In the case of LMCA thrombosis as well, subsequent stenting does not seem to expose the patient to a greater risk of subsequent thrombosis. It is quite likely that the vessel's large size, the presence of high flows and the vicinity to the aortic ostium are all factors favoring the low risk of stent thrombosis.

In the case of a large thrombus, attention should be paid to the possible pull-back of thrombotic material into the aorta along with the balloon used to pre-dilate and crush the clot or to deploy the stent, because of the risk of possible embolization phenomena (brain, etc). Therefore, before withdrawing the balloon, it is important to make sure that the guiding catheter is well cannulated in the LMCA and aspirate well any thrombotic debris from the Y-connector (Fig. 4.51).

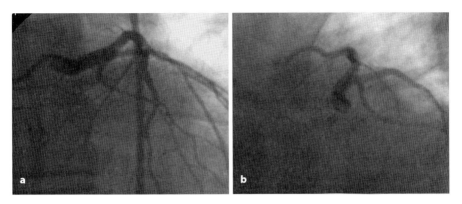

Fig 4.51 Thrombus in the ostial–proximal LMCA (**a**, **b**)

4.8.10
Dissection: Anterograde, Retrograde

This may occur following stent deployment, either because of failure to cover the entire plaque or as a result of the use of compliant or semi-compliant balloons for post-dilatation. In cases of major dissections limiting coronary flow, treatment envisages the implantation of another stent overlapping the prior one.

4.9
Intra-aortic Balloon Pump

Although desired by many [162], in actual fact, the intra-aortic balloon pump (IABP) has proven of great use only in some selected cases. As already stated above, simply passing the guidewires and pre-dilating again ensures a diameter and flow such that the procedure can proceed safely. An emergency patient with low cardiac output is another case, but, here too, the time needed to place an IABP can be beneficially used for rapid LMCA PCI. In these cases, the help of another operator can be useful, but what is even more useful is anesthesiological support with inotropic drugs and the infusion of fluids, which can adequately support cardiac output for the time needed to perform the procedure, and provide enough diastolic pressure to allow at least coronary artery pre-dilatation. This is the strategy usually adopted by our team in daily practice to tackle these emergency situations in LMCA treatment.

In the case of RCA disease and foreseeing a long-lasting, complex, procedure, IABP is to be recommended.

Periprocedural complications are a case of their own. In the case of LCX distal dissection in which it is impossible to cross the vessel with a balloon and/or stent, providing a high diastolic pressure is an essential prerequisite to cut the risk of vessel thrombosis or occlusion. In our experience, reopening and complete flow recovery has been achieved in both cases thanks to IABP (Fig. 4.52).

If instability persists following the procedure, IABP is recommended.

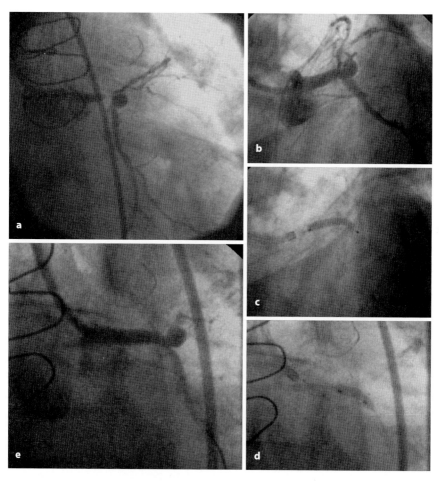

Fig. 4.52 Clinical case of LMCA bifurcation and periprocedural IABP use. **a** Distal subocclusive stenosis of protected LMCA. **b** After pre-dilatation and **c** after LMCA–LCX deployment and implantation of Carbostent (3.5/19 mm). **d** In-stent post-dilatation. (*cont.* ➤)

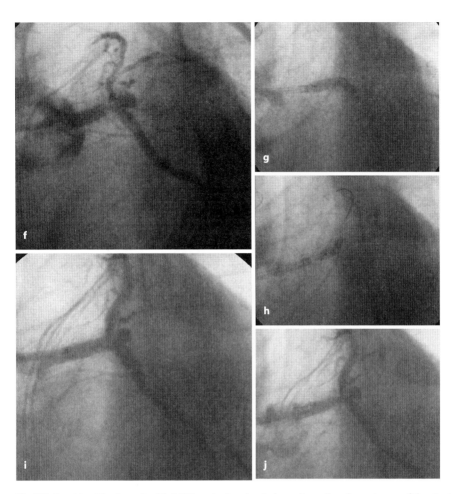

Fig. 4.52 (*cont.*) **e** Final result with LCX occlusion due to long dissection downstream of the stent. **f** Angiographic follow-up at 6 months: recurrence of flow in the LCX, critical in-stent stenosis. **g, h** In-stent dilatation. **i** Placement of stent (Taxus 3.5/16 mm) in-stent. **j** Final result

4.10
Specific Anatomical Scenarios

4.10.1
Left Main Coronary Artery Trifurcation

LMCA trifurcation lesions are technically even more challenging, with the potential for both early procedural complications (stent distortion, plaque shift, dissection, SB trapping) and late ISR. Part of the complexity of treating this subset of lesions relates to the different anatomic patterns of the stenosis, given the possible involvement of the proximal and distal part of the MB and/or the SBs, the close proximity of SBs' origin, the angle of SB take-off and the size of both the MB and SBs. Anatomically, trifurcation is defined as a close origin of two SBs from the MB, identified as the distance of both the SB take-off <3mm and a branch size of at least 2.25 mm at baseline angiography or after predilation. Trifurcation lesion is defined as a diameter of stenosis >50% within 5 mm from the carina involving the MB, associated or not with significant disease in either one or both SBs. The MB is defined as the larger branch with the largest perfusion territory. Between two SBs, the one with the narrowest angle from the distal MB is defined as SB1. It is important when choosing the treatment strategy to evaluate the four different angles of trifurcation and the size of carina (Figs. 4.22, 4.23). According to vessel anatomy, lesion distribution (e.g. SBs significantly narrowed at the ostium or within few millimiters) and/or when a significant plaque shift is expected, the operator can decide to implant three, two or one stent, such as in the common technique for bifurcation lesion (T-provisional, crush, minicrush, V-stenting, T-modified, provisional T stenting).

4.10.2
Stenosis of Both the Right Coronary Artery and the Left Main Coronary Artery

There are situations in which, alongside a critical LMCA lesion, RCA stenosis is also present. Analysis of our registry's data has shown that residual RCA disease is a determinant of adverse outcome following LMCA PCI. The objective of complete revascularization should hence always be pursued, as reported [163]. However, from a purely technical viewpoint, a diseased RCA does not lead to an increase in intrahospital complications. In this case as well, with the aid of appropriate expedients, which vary case by case, PCI can be performed.

4.10.2.1
Occluded Right Coronary Artery

This case requires that procedure time be reduced to the minimum, in order to minimize ischemia time, hence avoiding episodes of low cardiac output. In cases in which the RCA receives heterocoronary collaterals from the left coronary artery and shows a morphological pattern that is treatable by PCI in a short time and without any need for specific technical expedients, an attempt to open the RCA can be made before LMCA treatment in the presence of clinically stable conditions. Otherwise it is recommended to treat the LMCA lesion and schedule RCA de-obstruction in a later session. In the first case, once the coronary guidewire to the LAD edge (preferable) or LCX edge is deployed, also with the guiding catheter in a semi-selective position, lesion pre-dilatation can ensure adequate flow and allow PCI in safe conditions. If difficulties are encountered in crossing the lesion with the guidewire, it is recommended not to proceed any further and to make another attempt with a hydrophilic guidewire in order to prevent possible lesion destabilization and dramatic acute thrombosis. In our experience, the in-hospital mortality of 33 patients with occluded RCA treated with PCI amounted to 3%.

4.10.2.2
Diseased Right Coronary Artery

In this case the choice of the PCI method and timing varies depending on the case and operator experience. A series of assessments is needed to choose the right strategy:

- if the operator is not very experienced, a strategy envisages simultaneous semi-selective cannulation of both coronary ostia. This ensures rapid treatment of the LMCA lesion if there is a procedural difficulty or destabilized clinical conditions during RCA treatment. In this case, after cannulation of the ostia and deployment of a coronary guidewire in the left coronary artery, the RCA lesion is treated with the left guiding catheter in a semi-selective position, and then the LMCA can be treated in more stable conditions. In our experience, double engagement of the coronary artery ostia has been performed in a case of diseased ostia and a case of retrograde and anterograde LMCA de-obstruction in a patient already treated with two coronary artery bypass grafts in whom the grafts were occluded and the only patent one was stenosed
- if the right coronary artery provides a collateral for the left, the choice is to be made based on the overall angiographic assessment, the back-up of the guiding catheter in the two ostia, and the type, extent, and site of the lesion in the RCA and LMCA.

In any case, in general, before treating LMCA bifurcation, it is recommended to ensure patency of the RCA. If the RCA provides a collateral for the left side and is affected by non-severe stenosis with stable plaque, the LMCA can be treated first, followed by the RCA. This can be useful in the event of technical difficulties occurring during LMCA treatment. In this case the patient can be sent for complete surgical revascularization without incurring thrombosis of the stent already implanted in the RCA.

The aforementioned considerations are not of primary importance when treating lesions affecting the LMCA ostium and shaft, which are technically simple to treat also, regardless of whether or not the RCA is diseased.

If the LMCA provides a collateral for the RCA and the LMCA lesion is not tight, the RCA can be treated first, followed by the LMCA. One alternative that is always viable is double cannulation of the ostia, deployment of the guidewires, and subsequent treatment of the easier lesion, while remaining prepared to immediately treat the LMCA lesion.

Thrombosis and Antiplatelet Therapy

5

The use of DES has substantially reduced restenosis and expanded the frontiers of coronary angioplasty, allowing the effective treatment of increasingly complex lesions, which were previously considered to require surgery. However, the use of DES has recently been at the center of various controversies relating to an associated potential increase in thrombosis owing to delayed DES endothelialization. Thrombosis is an extremely relevant phenomenon when dealing with a vessel of critical importance like the LMCA, as the consequences of a thrombotic event can prove to be catastrophic. Various reports of patients with LMCA disease treated with DES have shown that thrombosis occurs with a very low frequency. Studies on LMCA PCI with DES have reported a total incidence of definite and probable thrombosis (including early, late, and very late thrombosis), as defined by the Academic Research Consortium (ARC), of no more than 1% [52, 64, 65]. In particular, very late definite thrombosis is seldom observed, with a reported frequency ranging between 0% and 0.3% [52, 64, 65]. A more recent study specifically assessed the incidence of thrombosis according to ARC definitions in 731 patients affected by LMCA stenosis treated with SES or PES in five centers [164]. Definite or probable thrombosis was observed in 0.95% of the study population at 2.5 years. All these thrombotic events affected the LMCA bifurcation, which, in the majority of cases, was treated with the two-stent technique. No cases of very late definite thrombosis were observed. Probable thrombosis was observed in 20 patients (2.7%), 8 (40%) of whom were still receiving double antiplatelet therapy. Moreover, it should be noted that 40% of patients were aged over 75 years, and 65% had an EF of less than 40% and a Euroscore of ≥6. Another important aspect is that all cases of definite and probable thrombosis occurred during the period of double antiplatelet therapy, thus suggesting the possible determining role of inadequate response to clopidogrel, rather than stent failure [164].

The existence of a potential risk of stent thrombosis has underscored the crucial role of double antiplatelet therapy with aspirin and clopidogrel, which the current guidelines recommend for a period of at least 12 months following the procedure [165]. Since LMCA is a highly critical site with the highest risk, continuing antiplatelet therapy for more than a year and even indefinitely has been suggested. This strategy, albeit seemingly prudent, does not appear to be warranted and supported by evidence, considering the extremely low occurrence of very late LMCA thrombosis (near 0%), the considerable potential risk of bleeding, and the high costs associated with prolonged antiplatelet therapy.

There is increasing evidence that, despite the proven benefits of clopidogrel, a substantial number of patients still have thrombotic events. In a recent substudy of the SICI-GISE survey on ULMCA stenosis, it was observed that the risk of cardiac mortality and myocardial infarction while on dual antiplatelet therapy is concentrated in the first 6 months after stenting, prompting the development of new therapeutic strategies reducing the risk in this specific time interval [166]. The occurrence of thrombotic events while patients are still taking aspirin and clopidogrel has been partly ascribed to an inadequate level of platelet inhibition in response to clopidogrel, warranting the need for more intense antiplatelet regimes. A wide range of variability has been observed in the degree of blocking of $P2Y_{12}$ (site of action of thienopyridines) induced by clopidogrel [167]. These patients maintaining a high level of platelet reactivity despite clopidogrel therapy are defined "clopidogrel non-responders", and they show a higher risk of thrombotic events [167]. Resistance to clopidogrel is a multifactorial phenomenon in which genetic, cellular, and clinical factors are all possible mechanisms [167]. Considering its major clinical implications, achieving optimal management of non-responders is imperative, although it is still quite unclear at the moment. An initial approach consists of fixing the modifiable clinical factors that can cause inadequate response, such as the lipid and glucose levels, arterial blood pressure, and the interaction with other drugs (possible interaction with statins and omeprazole). Based on the concept that clopidogrel under-dosing may be a key factor in determining clopidogrel responsiveness, one suggested strategy to improve the response to clopidogrel consists of increasing both the loading dose and maintenance dose. In functional trials, a 600 mg loading dose has been associated with earlier, greater, and longer platelet inhibition compared to the 300 mg standard dose [168, 169]. In addition, pilot studies have shown that a higher loading dose is associated with better clinical outcomes [169, 170]. A maintenance dose of 150 mg has been associated in several platelet function tests with a higher degree of platelet inhibition compared to the 75 mg standard dose of clopidogrel [171–173]. The guidelines [46] clearly state that "in patients in whom thrombosis may be catastrophic or lethal (ULMCA and LMCA bifurcation) platelet aggregation tests can be considered and the clopidogrel dose can be increased to 150 mg a day if platelet inhibition amounts to less than 50%" (Class IIb, level of evidence C). The latter statement also suggests an important major role for platelet function tests in clinical practice in order to optimize and customize anti-thrombotic therapy regimens [174]. It should be noted that studies reporting the functional effects of higher clopidogrel doses have shown that there is still a high percentage of non-responders despite the increase in dose [168, 172, 173]. This suggests a need for more powerful selective $P2Y_{12}$ inhibitors or alternative anti-thrombotic regimens [175]. New oral $P2Y_{12}$ antagonists are being studied, among which prasugrel is the one in the most advanced stage of investigation. Prasugrel, compared to clopidogrel, gives faster and more intense platelet inhibition and hence a lower variability in response. Greater platelet inhibition gives a better clinical outcome in patients with high thrombotic risk undergoing stenting, as reported in TRITON-TIMI 38 [176]. Antiplatelet drugs inhibiting targets other than $P2Y_{12}$ and in particular, the thrombin receptor, are also being investigated. Phase III trials are assessing the clinical efficacy of SCH530348 and E5555, two oral reversible PAR-1 inhibitors (thrombin protease-activated receptor), in addition to standard double anti-platelet therapy with aspirin and clopidogrel. In a subanalysis of the GISE-SICI registry evaluating the impact of acute coronary syndrome (ACS) on outcomes after DES implantation in ULMCA, it was shown that, during 2-year follow up, the adjusted HR of cardiac mortality and myocardial infarction of patients with ACS ($n = 611$) versus stable patients ($n = 490$) was 2.42 (95% CI 1.37–4.28; $P = 0.002$) [177]. Of note, a gradient of increased risk moving from stable patients to unstable patients with non-ST-segment elevation acute myocardial infarction was observed. This increased risk associated with ACS was concentrated in the first year after DES implantation, while thereafter patients with ACS had similar outcomes to stable patients [177]. This finding of a negative impact of ACS underscores the need for individualized and more powerful antiplatelet regimes in particularly high-risk clinical settings, such as during the first year after DES implantation in the LMCA in the context of an ACS.

In conclusion, the optimization of anti-thrombotic therapy as an essential pharmacological support to LMCA PCI further contributes to minimizing the clinical risks of this strategy for treatment, which has proven to be technically safe and efficacious in both the medium and long term.

References

1. Thomas M, Hildick-Smith D, Louvard Y et al. Percutaneous coronary intervention for bifurcation disease. A consensus view from the first meeting of the European Bifurcation Club. Eurointervention 2006;2:149–153.
2. De Lezo JS, Medina A, Romero M et al. Predictors of restenosis following unprotected left coronary stenting. Am J Cardiol 2001;88:308–310.
3. Alexander RW, Griffith GL. Anomalies of the coronary arteries and their clinical significance. Circulation 1956;14:800–805.
4. Hauser M. Congenital anomalies of the coronary arteries. Heart 2005;91:1240–1245.
5. Taylor AJ, Virmani R. coronary artery anomalies in adults: which are high risk? ACC Curr J Rev 2001;10:92–94.
6. Palmieri C. Atlante delle anomalie coronariche. Primula Multimedia Editore 2005;50–51.
7. Proudfit WL, Shirey EK, Sones FM. Distribution of arterial lesions demonstrated by selective cinecoronary arteriography. Circulation 1967;36:54–62.
8. Fischer M, Mayer B, Baessler A et al. Familial aggregation of left main coronary artery disease and future risk of coronary events in asymptomatic siblings of affected patients. Eur Heart J 2007;28:2432–2437.
9. Gazetopoulos N, Ioannidis PJ, Karydis C et al. Short left coronary artery trunk as a risk factor in the development of coronary atherosclerosis. Pathological study. Br Heart J 1976;38:1160–1165.
10. Cameron A, Kemp HG, Fisher LD et al. Left main coronary artery stenosis: angiographic determination. Circulation 1983;68:484–489.
11. Wang JC, Normand SL, Mauri L, Kuntz RE. Coronary artery spatial distribution of acute myocardial infarction occlusions. Circulation 2004;110:278–284.
12. Valgimigli M, Gastón A, Rodriguez-Granillo GA et al. Plaque composition in the left main stem mimics the distal but not the proximal tract of the left coronary artery J Am Coll Cardiol 2007;49:23–31.
13. Rodriguez-Granillo GA, Garcia-Garcia HM, Wentzel J et al. Plaque composition and its relationship with acknowledged shear stress patterns in coronary arteries. J Am Coll Cardiol 2006;47:884–885.
14. Hartnell GG, Parnell BM, Pride RB. Coronary artery ectasia: its prevalence and clinical significance in 4993 patients. Br Heart J 1985;54:392–395.

15. Swaye PS, Fisher LD, Litwin P et al. Aneurysmal coronary artery disease. Circulation 1983;67:134–138.

16. Topaz O, Di Sciascio G, Cowley MJ et al. Angiographic features of left main coronary artery. Am J Cardiol 1991;67:1139–1142.

17. Syed M, Lesch M. Coronary artery aneurysm: a review. Prog Cardiovasc Dis 1997;40:77–84.

18. Smith MD, Cowley MJ, Vetrovec GW. Aneurysms of the left main coronary artery: a report of three cases and review of the literature. Cathet Cardiovasc Diagn 1984;10:583–591.

19. Tunick PA, Slater J, Kronzon I, Glassman E. Discrete atherosclerotic coronary artery aneurysms: a study of 20 patients. J Am Coll Cardiol 1990;15:279–282.

20. Rahmatullah SI, Khan IA, Nair VM et al. Bifurcating aneurysm of left main coronary artery involving left anterior descending and left circumflex arteries. Angiology 1999;50:417–420.

21. Robertson T, Fisher L. Prognostic significance of coronary artery aneurysm and ectasia in the coronary Artery Surgery Study (CASS) registry. Prog Clin Biol Res 1987;250:325–339.

22. Hill JA, Margolis JR, Feldman RL et al. Coronary arterial aneurysm formation after balloon angioplasty. Am J Cardiol 1983;52:261–264.

23. De Cesare NB, Popma JJ, Holmes DR Jr et al. Clinical angiographic and histologic correlates of ectasia after directional coronary atherectomy. Am J Cardiol 1992;69:314–319.

24. Jorgensen MB, Aharonian V, Mansukhani P, Mahrer PR. Spontaneous coronary dissection: a cluster of cases with this rare finding. Am Heart J 1994;127:1382–1387.

25. Auer J, Punzengruber C, Weber T et al. Spontaneous coronary artery dissection involving the left main stem: assessment by intravascular ultrasound. Heart 2004;90:e39.

26. Conraads VM, Vorlat A, Colpaert CG et al. Spontaneous dissection of three major coronary arteries subsequent to cystic medial necrosis. Chest 1999;116:1473–1475.

27. Chahine RA, Raizner AE, Ishimori T et al. The incidence and clinical implications of coronary artery spasm. Circulation 1975; 52: 972–978.

28. Tzivoni D, Merin G, Milo S, Gotsman MS. Spasm of left main coronary artery. Br Heart J 1976;38:104–107.

29. Takaro T, Ultgren HN, Lipton MJ, Detre KM. The VA cooperative randomized study of surgery for coronary artery occlusive disease II. Subgroup with significant left main lesions. Circulation 1976;3:107–117.

30. Varnauskas E, for the European Coronary Sugery Study Group.Twelve-year follow-up of survival in the randomized European Coronary Sugery Study. N Engl J Med 1988;319:332–337.

31. Caracciolo EA, Davis KB, Sopko G et al. Comparison of surgical and medical group survival in patients with left main equivalent coronary artery disease: long-term CASS experience. Circulation 1995;91:2335–2344.

32. Keogh BE, Kinsman R. Fifth National Adult Cardiac Surgical Database Report 2003. Dendrite Clinical Systems, Henley-on-Thames, 2004.

33. Yeatman M, Caputo M, Ascione R et al. Off-pump coronary artery bypass surgery for critical left main stem disease: safety, efficacy and outcome. Eur J Cardiothorac Surg 2001;19:239–244.

34. Lu JC, Grayson AD, Pullan DM. On-pump versus off-pump surgical revascularization for left main stem stenosis: risk adjusted outcomes. Ann Thorac Surg 2005;80:136–142.
35. Dewey TM, Magee MJ, Edgerton JR et al. Off-pump bypass grafting is safe in patients with left main coronary disease. Ann Thorac Surg 2001;72:788–791.
36. Ellis SG, Hill CM, Lytle BW. Spectrum of surgical risk for left main coronary stenoses: benchmark for potentially competing percutaneous therapies. Am Heart J 1998;135:335–338.
37. Jonsson A, Hammar N, Nordquist T, Ivert T. Left main coronary artery stenosis no longer a risk factor for early and late death after coronary artery bypass surgery – an experience covering three decades. Eur J Cardiothorac Surg 2006;30:311–317.
38. Grüntzig AR, Senning A, Siegenthaler W. Nonoperative dilatation of coronary-artery stenosis. Percutaneous transluminal coronary angioplasty. N Engl J Med 1979;301:61–68.
39. O'Keefe JH Jr, Hartzler GO, Rutherford BD et al. Left main coronary angioplasty: early and late results of 127 acute and elective procedures. Am J Cardiol 1989;64:144–147.
40. Silvestri M, Barragan P, Sainsous J et al. Unprotected left main coronary artery stenting: immediate and medium-term outcomes of 140 elective procedures. J Am Coll Cardiol 2000;35:1543–1550.
41. Tan WA, Tamai H, Park SJ et al. Long-term clinical outcomes after unprotected left main trunk percutaneous revascularization in 279 patients. Circulation 2001;104:1609–1614.
42. Black A, Cortina R, Bossi I et al. Unprotected left main coronary artery stenting: correlates of midterm survival and impact of patient selection. J Am Coll Cardiol 2001;37:832–838.
43. Takagi T, Stankovic G, Finci L et al. Results and long-term predictors of adverse clinical events after elective percutaneous interventions on unprotected left main coronary artery. Circulation 2002;106:698–702.
44. Park SJ, Park SW, Hong MK et al. Long-term (three-year) outcomes after stenting of unprotected left main coronary artery stenosis in patients with normal left ventricular function. Am J Cardiol 2003;91:12–16.
45. Silber S, Albertsson P, Aviles FF et al. Guidelines for percutaneous coronary interventions: The Task Force for Percutaneous Coronary Interventions of the European Society of Cardiology. Eur Heart J 2005;26:804–847.
46. Smith SC Jr, Feldman TE, Hirshfeld JW Jr et al. ACC/AHA/SCAI 2005 guideline update for percutaneous coronary intervention: summary article: a report of the American College of Cardiology/American Heart Association Task Force on Practice Guidelines (ACC/AHA/SCAI Writing Committee to Update the 2001 Guidelines for Percutaneous Coronary Intervention). Circulation 2006;113:156–175.
47. Rao SV, Shaw RE, Brindis RG et al. On- versus off-label use of drug-eluting coronary stents in clinical practice (report from the American College of Cardiology National Cardiovascular Data Registry (NCDR)). Am J Cardiol 2006;97:1478–1481.
48. De Lezo JS, Medina A, Pan M et al. Rapamycin-eluting stents for the treatment of unprotected left main coronary disease. Am Heart J 2004;148:481–485.
49. Migliorini A, Moschi G, Giurlani L et al. Drug-eluting stent supported percutaneous coronary intervention for unprotected left main disease. Catheter Cardiovasc Interv 2006;68:225–230.

50. Agostoni P, Valgimigli M, Van Mieghem CA et al. Comparison of early outcome of percutaneous coronary intervention for unprotected left main coronary artery disease in the drug-eluting stent era with versus without intravascular ultrasonic guidance. Am J Cardiol 2005;95:644–647.

51. Vecchio S, Chechi T, Vittorio G et al. Outlook of drug-cluting stent implantation for unprotected left main disease: insights on long term clinical predictor. J Invasive Cardiol 2007;19:388–389.

52. Sheiban I, Meliga E, Moretti C et al. Long-term clinical and angiographic outcomes of treatment of unprotected left main artery stenosis with sirolimus-eluting stent. Am J Cardiol 2007;100:431–435.

53. Valgimigli M, van Mieghem CA, Ong ATL et al. Short- and long-term clinical outcome after drug-eluting stent implantation for the percutaneous treatment of left main coronary artery disease: Insights from the Rapamycin-Eluting and Taxus Stent Evaluated at Rotterdam Cardiology Hospital (RESEARCH and T-SEARCH) registries. 2005;111:1383–1389.

54. Park SJ, Kim YH, Lee BK et al. Sirolimus-eluting stent implantation for unprotected left main coronary artery stenosis: comparison with bare metal stent implantation. J Am Coll Cardiol 2005;45:351–356.

55. Chieffo A, Stankovic G, Bonizzoni E et al. Early and mid-term results of drug-eluting stent implantation in unprotected left main. Circulation 2005;111:791–795.

56. Sheiban I, Meliga E, Moretti C et al. Sirolimus-eluting stents vs. bare metal stents for the treatment of unprotected left main coronary artery stenosis. Eurointervention 2006;2:356–362.

57. Gao RL, Xu B, Chen JL et al. Immediate and long-term outcomes of drug-eluting stent implantation for unprotected left main coronary artery disease: comparison with bare-metal stent implantation Am Heart J 2008;55:553–561.

58. Palmerini T, Marzocchi A, Marrozzini C et al. Comparison between coronary angio-plasty and coronary bypass surgery for the treatment of unprotected left main coronary artery stenosis. Am J Cardiol 2006;98:54–59.

59. Lee MS, Kapoor N, Jamal F et al. Comparison of coronary artery bypass surgery with percutaneous coronary intervention with drug-eluting stents for unprotected left main coronary artery disease. J Am Coll Cardiol 2006;47:864–870.

60. Chieffo A, Morici N, Maisano F et al. Percutaneous treatment with drug eluting stent implantation versus bypass surgery for unprotected left main stenosis. A single center experience. Circulation 2006;113:2542–2547.

61. Sanmartin M, Baz JA, Claro R et al. Comparison of drug-eluting stents versus surgery for unprotected left main coronary artery disease. Am J Cardiol 2007;100:970–973.

62. Biondi-Zoccai GG, Lotrionte M, Moretti C et al. A collaborative systematic review and meta-analysis on 1278 patiets undergoing percutaneous drug-eluting stenting for unpro-tected left main coronary artery disesase. Am Heart J 2008;155:274–283.

63. Valgimigli M, Malagutti P, Aoki J et al. Sirolimus-eluting versus paclitaxel-eluting stent implantation for the percutaneous treatment of left main coronary artery disease: a combined RESEARCH and T-SEARCH long term analysis. J Am Coll Cardiol 2006;47:507–514.

64. Tamburino C, Angiolillo DJ, Capranzano P et al. Long-term clinical outcomes after drug-eluting stent implantation in unprotected left main coronary artery disease. Catheter Cardiovasc Interv 2009;73:291–298.

65. Meliga E, Garcia-Garcia HM, Valgimigli M et al. Longest available clinical outcomes after drug-eluting stent implantation for unprotected left main coronary artery disease The DELFT (Drug Eluting stent for LeFT main) registry. J Am Coll Cardiol 2008;51:2212–2219.

66. Palmerini T, Marzocchi A, Tamburino C et al. Two-year clinical outcome with drug-eluting stents versus bare-metal stents in a real world registry of unprotected left main coronary artery stenosis from the Italian Sociery of Invasive Cardiology. Am J Cardiol 2008;102:1463–1468.

67. Seung KB, Park DW, Kim YH et al. Stents versus coronary-artery bypass grafting for the left main coronary artery disease. N Engl J Med 2008;358:1781–1792.

68. Brener SJ, Galla JM, Bryant III R et al. Comparison of percutaneous versus surgical revascularization of severe unprotected left main coronary stenosis in matched patients. Am J Cardiol 2008;101:169–172.

69. Tamburino C, Di Salvo ME, Capodanno D et al. Comparison of drug-eluting stents and bare-metal stents for the treatment of unprotected left main coronary artery disease in acute coronary syndromes. Am J Cardiol 2009;103:187–193.

70. Capodanno D, Di Salvo ME, Palmerini T et al. Long-term clinical benefit of drug-eluting stents over bare-metal stents in diabetic patients with de novo left main coronary artery disease. Results from a real-world multicenter registry. Catheter Cardiovasc Interv 2009;73:310–316.

71. Palmerini T, Barlocco F, Santarelli A et al. A comparison between coronary artery bypass grafting surgery and drug eluting stent for the treatment of unprotected left main coronary artery disease in elderly patients (aged ≥75 years). Eur Heart J 2007;28:2714–2719.

72. Rodés-Cabau J, DeBlois J, Bertrand OF et al. Nonrandomized comparison of coronary artery bypass surgery and percutaneous coronary intervention for the treatment of unprotected left main coronary artery disease in octogenarians. Circulation 2008;118:2374–2381.

73. Buszman P, Kiesz SR, Bochenek A et al. Acute and late outcomes of unprotected left main stenting in comparison with surgical revascularization. J Am Coll Cardiol 2008;51:538–545.

74. Serruys PW, Morice MC, Kappetein AP et al.; the SYNTAX Investigators. Percutaneous coronary intervention versus coronary-artery bypass grafting for severe coronary artery disease. N Engl J Med 2009;360:961–972.

75. Valgimigli M, Malagutti P, Rodriguez-Granillo GA et al. Distal left main coronary disease is a major predictor of outcome in patients undergoing percutaneous intervention in the drug-eluting stent era an integrated clinical and angiographic analysis based on the Rapamycin-Eluting Stent Evaluated At Rotterdam Cardiology Hospital (RESEARCH) and Taxus-Stent Evaluated At Rotterdam Cardiology Hospital (T-SEARCH) Registries. J Am Coll Cardiol 2006;47:1530–1537.

76. Meliga E, Garcia-Garcia HM, Valgimigli M et al. Impact of drug-eluting stent selection on long-term clinical outcomes in patients treated for unprotected left main coronary artery disease: the sirolimus vs paclitaxel drug-eluting stent for left main registry (SP-DELFT). Int J Cardiol 2008:5 August, Epub ahead of print.

77. Palmerini T, Marzocchi A, Tamburino C et al. Impact of bifurcation technique on 2-year clinical outcomes in 773 patients with distal unprotected left main coronary artery stenosis treated with drug-eluting stents. Circ Cardiovasc Intervent 2008;1:185–192.

78. Chieffo A, Park SJ, Valgimigli M et al. Favorable long-term outcome after drug-eluting stent implantation in nonbifurcation lesions that involve unprotected left main coronary artery. A multicenter registry. Circulation 2007;116:158–162.

79. Furuichi S, Sangiorgi GM, Palloshi A et al. Drug eluting stent implantation in coronary trifurcation lesion. J Invasive Cardiol 2007;19:284–285.

80. Shammas NW, Dippel EJ, Avilla A et al. Long term outcomes in treating of left main trifurcation coronary artery disease with the paclitaxel-eluting stent. J Invasive Cardiol 2007;19:77–82.

81. Sheiban I, Gerasimou A, Bollati M et al. Early and long-term results of percutaneous coronary intervention for unprotected left main trifurcation disease. Catheter Cardiovasc Interv 2009;73:25–31.

82. Tamburino C, Tomasello D, Capodanno D et al. Long term follow up after drug eluting stent implantation in left main trifurcation. Eurointervention 2009;in press.

83. Cameron A, Kemp HG Jr, Fisher LD et al. Left main coronary artery stenosis: angiographic determination. Circulation 1983;68:484–489.

84. Fisher LD, Judkins MP, Lesperance J et al. Reproducibility of coronary arteriographic reading in the coronary artery surgery study (CASS). Cathet Cardiovasc Diagn 1982;8:565–575.

85. Lindstaedt M, Spiecker M, Perings C et al. How good are experienced interventional cardiologists at predicting the functional significance of intermediate or equivocal left main coronary artery stenoses? Int J Cardiol 2007;20:254–261.

86. Boden WE, Ferguson TB Jr, Guyton RA et al. Revascularization for unprotected left main stem coronary artery stenosis stenting or surgery. J Am Coll Cardiol 2008;51:885–892.

87. Roy P, Steinberg DH, Sushinsky SJ et al. The potential clinical utility of intravascular ultrasound guidance in patients undergoing percutaneous coronary intervention with drug-eluting stents. Eur Heart J 2008;29:1851–1857.

88. Zhou Y, Kassab GS, Molloi S. On the design of the coronary arterial tree: a generalization of Murray's law. Phys Med Biol 1999;44:2929–2945.

89. Jasti V, Ivan E, Yalamanchili V et al. Correlations between fractional flow reserve and intravascular ultrasound in patients with an ambiguous left main coronary artery stenosis. Circulation 2004;110:2831–2836.

90. Park SJ, Hong MK, Lee CW et al. Elective stenting of unprotected left main coronary artery stenosis: effect of debulking before stenting and intravascular ultrasound guidance. J Am Coll Cardiol 2001;38:1054–1060.

91. Erglis A, Narbute I, Kumsars I et al. A randomized comparison of paclitaxel-eluting stents versus bare-metal stents for treatment of unprotected left main coronary artery stenosis. J Am Coll Cardiol 2007;50:491–497.

92. Pijls NH, De Bruyne B, Peels K et al. Measurement of fractional flow reserve to assess the functional severity of coronary artery stenoses. N Engl J Med 1996;334:1703–1738.

93. Bech GJ, De Bruyne B, Pijls NH et al. Fractional flow reserve to determine the appropriateness of angioplasty in moderate coronary stenosis: a randomized trial. Circulation 2001;103:2928–2933.

94. Berger A, Botman KJ, MacCarthy PA et al. Long-term clinical outcome after fractional flow reserve-guided percutaneous coronary intervention in patients with multivessel disease. J Am Coll Cardiol 2005;46:438–442.

95. Botman KJ, Pijls NH, Bech JW et al. Percutaneous coronary intervention or bypass surgery in multivessel disease? A tailored approach based on coronary pressure measurement. Catheter Cardiovasc Interv 2004;63:184–191.

96. Bech GJ, Droste H, Pijls NH et al. Value of fractional flow reserve in making decisions about bypass surgery for equivocal left main coronary artery disease. Heart 2001;86:547–552.

97. Jiménez-Navarro M, Hernández-García JM, Alonso-Briales JH et al. Should we treat patients with moderately severe stenosis of the left main coronary artery and negative FFR results. J Invasive Cardiol 2004;16:398–400.

98. Legutko J, Dudek D, Rzeszutko L et al. Fractional flow reserve assessment to determine the indications for myocardial revascularisation in patients with borderline stenosis of the left main coronary artery. Kardiol Pol 2005;63:499–506.

99. Suemaru S, Iwasaki K, Yamamoto K et al. Coronary pressure measurement to determine treatment strategy for equivocal left main coronary artery lesions. Heart Vessels 2005;20:271–277.

100. Lindstaedt M, Yazar A, Germing A et al. Clinical outcome in patients with intermediate or equivocal left main coronary artery disease after deferral of surgical revascularization on the basis of fractional flow reserve measurements. Am Heart J 2006;152:e1–9.

101. Koo BK, Kang HJ, Youn TJ et al. Physiologic assessment of jailed side branch lesions using fractional flow reserve. J Am Coll Cardiol 2005;46:633–637.

102. Stamper D, Weissman NJ, Brezinski M. Plaque characterization with optical coherence tomography. J Am Coll Cardiol 2006;47:C69–C79.

103. Matsumoto D, Shite J, Shinke T et al. Neointimal coverage of sirolimus-eluting stents at 6-month followup: evaluated by optical coherence tomography. Eur Heart J 2007;28:918–919.

104. Tearney GJ, Waxman S, Shishkov M et al. Three-dimensional coronary artery microscopy by intracoronary optical frequency domain imaging. J Am Coll Cardiol 2008;1:752–761.

105. Thomas AC, Davies MJ, Dilly S et al. Potential errors in the estimation of coronary arterial stenosis from clinical arteriography with reference to the shape of the coronary arterial lumen. Br Heart J 1968;55:129–139.

106. Katritsis D, Webb-Peploe M. Limitations of coronary angiography: an understimated problem? Clin Cardiol 1991;14:20–24.

107. Isner JM, Kishel J, Kent KM et al. Accuracy of angiographic determination of left main coronary arterial narrowing. Angiographic-histologic correlative analysis in 28 patients. Circulation 1981;63:1056–1064.

108. Dvir D, Marom H, Guetta V, Kornowski R. Three-dimensional coronary reconstruction from routine single-plane coronary angiograms: in vivo quantitative validation. Int J Cardiovasc Intervent 2005;7:141–145.

109. Gollapudi RR, Valencia R, Lee SS et al. Utility of threedimensional reconstruction of coronary angiographyto guide percutaneous coronary intervention. Catheter Cardiovasc Interven 2007;69:479–482.

110. Schlundt C, Kreft JG, Fuchs F et al. Three dimensional on line reconstruction of coronary bifurcated lesions to optimize side-branch stenting. Catheter Cardiovasc Interv 2006;68:249–253.

111. Gradaus R, Mathies K, Breithardt G, Bocker D. Clinical assessment of a new real time 3 D quantitative coronary angiography system: evaluation in stented vessel segments. Catheter Cardiovasc Interv 2006;68:44–49.

112. Dvir D, Marom H, Guetta V, Kornowski R. Three-dimensional coronary reconstruction from routine single-plane coronary angiograms: in vivo quantitative validation. Int J Cardiovasc Intervent 2005;7:141–145.

113. Abdulla J, Abildstrom SZ, Gotzsche O et al. 64-multislice detector computed tomography coronary angiography as potential alternative to conventional coronary angiography: a systematic review and meta-analysis. Eur Heart J 2007;28:3042–3050.

114. Hausleiter J, Meyer T, Hermann F et al. Estimated radiation dose associated with cardiac CT angiography. JAMA 2009;301:500–507.

115. Budoff MJ, Dowe D, Jollis JG et al. Diagnostic performance of 64-multidetector row coronary computer tomographic angiography for evaluation of coronary artery stenosis in individuals without known coronary artery disease: results from the prospective multicenter ACCURACY (Assessment by Coronary Computed Tomographic Angiography of Individuals Undergoing Invasive Coronary Angiography) trial. J Am Coll Cardiol 2008;52:1724–1732.

116. Mollet NR, Cademartiri F, van Mieghem CA et al. High-resolution spiral computed tomography coronary angiography in patients referred for diagnostic conventional coronary angiography. Circulation 2005;112:2318–2323.

117. Leber AW, Knez A, von Ziegler F et al. Quantification of obstructive and nonobstructive coronary lesions by 64-slice computed tomography: a comparative study with quantitative coronary angiography and intravascular ultrasound. J Am Coll Cardiol 2005;46:147–154.

118. Rodriguez-Granillo GA, Rosales MA, Degrossi E et al. Multislice CT coronary angiography for the detection of burden, morphology and distribution of atherosclerotic plaques in the left main bifurcation. Int J Cardiovasc Imaging 2007;23:389–392.

119. Van Mieghem CA, Cademartiri F, Mollet NR et al. Multislice spiral computed tomography for the evaluation of stent patency after left main coronary artery stenting: a comparison with conventional coronary angiography and intravascular ultrasound. Circulation 2006;114:645–653.

120. Cordeiro MA, Lima JA. Atherosclerotic plaque characterization by multidetector row computed tomography angiography. J Am Coll Cardiol 2006;47(Suppl 8):C40–47.

121. Wilensky RL, Song HK, Ferrari VA. Role of magnetic resonance and intravascular magnetic resonance in the detection of vulnerable plaques. J Am Coll Cardiol 2006;47:C48–56.

122. Kim WY, Danias PG, Stuber M et al. Coronary magnetic resonance angiography for the detection of coronary stenoses. N Engl J Med 2001;345:1863–1869.

123. Sakuma H, Ichikawa Y, Chino S et al. Detection of coronary artery stenosis with whole-heart coronary magnetic resonance angiography. J Am Coll Cardiol 2006;48:1946–1950.

124. Kern MJ, Ouellette D, Frianeza T. A new technique to anchor stents for exact placement in ostial stenoses: the stent tail wire or Szabo technique. Catheter Cardiovasc Interv 2006;68:901–906.

125. Szabo S, Abramowitz B, Vaitkus PT. New technique for aorto-ostial stent placement. Am J Cardiol 2005;96:96H–212H.

126. Moses JW, Leon MB, Popma JJ et al. DIRECT: Direct stenting using the sirolimus-eluting Bx Velocity stent: procedural, clinical, and angiographic outcomes compared to a predilatation strategy. Paper presented at the American College of Cardiology 53rd Annual Scientific Session, New Orleans, LA, 7–10 March 2004.

127. Mehilli J, Kastrati A, Dirschinger J et al. Intracoronary stenting and angiographic results: restenosis after direct stenting versus stenting with predilation in patients with symptomatic coronary artery disease (ISAR-DIRECT Trial). Catheter Cardiovasc Interv 2004;61:190–195.

128. Brondie BR. Adjunctive balloon postdilatation after stent deployment: is it still necessary with drug-eluting stents? J Interv Cardiol 2006;19:43–50.

129. Brodie BR, Cooper C, Jones M et al.; Postdilatation Clinical Compartative Study (POSTIT) Investigators. Is adjunctive balloon post-dilatation necessary after coronary stent deployment? Final results from the POSTIT trial. Cathcter Cardiovasc Interv 2003;59:184–192.

130. Cheneau E, Satler LF, Escolar E et al. Underexpansion of sirolimus-eluting stents: Incidence and relationship to delivery pressure. Catheter Cardiovasc Interv 2005;65:222–226.

131. Blackman DJ, Porto I, Shirodaria C et al. Usefulness of high pressure post-dilatation to optimize deployment of drug-eluting stents for the treatment of diffuse instent coronary restenosis. Am J Cardiol 2004;94:922–925.

132. Tamburino C, Di Salvo ME, Capodanno D et al. Are drug eluting stents superior to bare metal stents in patients with unprotected non bifurcational left main disease? Insights from a multicenter registry. Eur Heart Journal 2009;in press.

133. Laham RJ, Carrozza JP, Baim DS. Treatment of unprotected left main stenoses with Palmaz- Shatz stenting. Cathet Cardiovasc Diagn 1996;37:77–80.

134. Fischell TA, Malhotra S, Khan S. A new ostial stent positioning system (Ostial Pro) for the accurate placement of stents to treat aorto-ostial lesions. Catheter Cardiovasc Interv 2008;71:353–357.

135. Laird JR. The SQUARE ONE stent: delivery systems and stents for coronary and peripheral ostial placement (BOSS-1; BullsEye Ostial Stent Study). Paper presented at the Transcatheter Cardiovascular Therapeutics 20th Annual Scientific Symposium, Washington, DC, 12–17 October 2008.

136. Louvard Y, Thomas M, Dzavik V et al. Classification of coronary artery bifurcation lesions and treatments: time for a consensus! Catheter Cardiovasc Interv 2008;71:175–183.

137. Medina A, Suarez de Lezo J, Pan M. A new classification of coronary bifurcation lesions. Rev Esp Cardiol 2006;59:183.

138. Cutlip DE, Baim DS, Ho KKL et al. Stent thrombosis in the modern era. A pooled analysis of multicenter coronary stent clinical trials. Circulation 2001;103:1967–1971.

139. Moreno R, Fernandez C, Hernandez R et al. Drug eluting stent thrombosis: results from a pooled analysis including 10 randomized studies. J Am Coll Cardiol 2005;45:954–959.

140. Orford JL, Lennon R, Melby S et al. Frequency and correlates of coronary stent thrombosis in the modern era. Analysis of a single center registry. J Am Coll Cardiol 2002;40:1567–1572.

141. Chieffo A, Bonizzoni E, Orlic D et al. Intraprocedural stent thrombosis during implantation of sirolimus-eluting stents. Circulation 2004;109:2732–2736.

142. Ong ATL, Hoye A, Aoki J et al. Thirty-day incidence and six-month clinical outcome of thrombotic stent occlusion after bare-metal, sirolimus, or paclitaxel stent implantation. J Am Coll Cardiol 2005;5:947–953.

143. Iakovou I, Schmidt T, Bonizzoni E et al. Incidence, predictors, and outcome of thrombosis after successful implantation of drug eluting stent. JAMA 2005;293:2126–2130.

144. Brunel P, Lefevre T, Darremont O, Louvard Y. Provisional T-stenting and kissing balloon in the treatment of coronary bifurcation lesions: Results of the French multicenter "TULIPE"study. Catheter Cardiovasc Interv 2006;68:67–73.

145. Alberti A, Missiroli B, Nannini C. "Skirt" technique for coronary artery bifurcation stenting. J Invasive Cardiol 2000;12:633–636.

146. Kobayashi Y, Colombo A, Adamian M et al. The skirt technique: a stenting technique to treat a lesion immediately proximal to the bifurcation (pseudobifurcation). Catheter Cardiovasc Interv 2000;51:347–351.

147. Cilingiroglu M, Elliott J, Patel D et al. Long-term effects of novel biolimus eluting DEVAX AXXESS plus nitinol self expanding stent in a porcine coronary model. Catheter Cardiovasc Interv 2006;68:271–289.

148. Chen J, Li JJ, Chen JL et al. Drug-eluting stents for the treatment of ostial coronary lesions: comparison of sirolimus-eluting stent with paclitaxel-eluting stent. Coron Artery Dis 2008;7:507–511.

149. Steigen TK, Maeng M, Wiseth R et al.; Nordic PCI Study Group. Randomized study on simple versus complex stenting of coronary artery bifurcation lesions: the Nordic bifurcation study. Circulation 2006;114:1955–1961.

150. Carrie D, Karouny E, Chouairi S, Puel J. T-shaped stent placement: a technique for the treatment of dissected bifurcation lesions. Cathet Cardiovasc Diagn 1996;37:311–313.

151. Kobayashi Y, Colombo A, Akiyama T et al. Modified "T" stenting: a technique for kissing stents in bifurcational coronarylesion. Cathet Cardiovasc Diagn 1998;43:323–326.

152. Porto I, van Gaal W, Banning A. "Crush" and "reverse crush" technique to treat a complex left main stenosis. Heart 2006;92:1021.

153. Galassi AR, Colombo A, Buchbinder M et al. Long-term outcomes of bifurcation lesions after implantation of drug-eluting stents with the "mini-crush technique". Catheter Cardiovasc Interv 2007;69:976–983.

154. Chevalier B, Glatt B, Royer T, Guyon P. Placement of coronary stents in bifurcation lesions by the "coulotte" technique. Am J Cardiol 1998;82:943–949.

155. Schampaert E, Fort S, Adelman AG, Schwartz L. The V-stent: a novel technique for coronary bifurcation stenting. Cathet Cardiovasc Diagn 1996;39:320–326.

156. Colombo A, Gaglione A, Nakamura S, Finci L. "Kissing" stents for bifurcational coronary lesion. Cathet Cardiovasc Diagn 1993;30:327–330.

157. Sharma SK. Simultaneous kissing drug-eluting stent technique for percutaneous treatment of bifurcation lesions in large-size vessels. Catheter Cardiovasc Interv 2005;65:10–16.

158. Sharma SK, Choudhury A, Lee J et al. Simultaneous kissing stents (SKS) technique for treating bifurcation lesions in medium-to large size coronary arteries. Am J Cardiol 2004;94:913–917.

159. Lefèvre T, Louvard Y, Morice MC et al. Stenting of bifurcation lesions: classification, treatments, and results. Catheter Cardiovasc Interv 2000;49:274–283.

160. Burzotta F, Gwon HC, Hahn JY et al. Modified T-stenting with intentional protrusion of the side-branch stent within the main vessel stent to ensure ostial coverage and facilitate final kissing balloon: the T-stenting and small protrusion technique (TAP-stenting). Report of bench testing and first clinical Italian-korean two-centre experience. Catheter Cardiovasc Interv 2007;70:75–82.

161. Sianos G, Vaina S, Hoye A, Serruys PW. Bifurcation stenting with drug eluting stents: Illustration of the Crush technique. Catheter Cardiovasc Interv 2006;67:839–845.

162. Briguori C, Airoldi F, Chieffo A et al. Elective versus provisional intraaortic balloon pumping in unprotected left main stenting. Am Heart J 2006;152:565–572.

163. Tamburino C, Angiolillo DJ, Capranzano P et al. Complete versus incomplete revascularization in patients with multivessel disease undergoing percutaneous coronary intervention with drug-eluting stents. Catheter Cardiovasc Interv 2008;72:448–456.

164. Chieffo A, Park SJ, Meliga E et al. Late and very late stent trombosis following drug-eluting stent implantation in unprotected left main coronary artery: a multicentre registry. Eur Heart J 2008;29:2108–2115.

165. King SB 3rd, Smith SC Jr, Hirshfeld JW Jr et al. 2007 focused update of the ACC/AHA/SCAI 2005 guideline update for percuteneous coronary intervention: a report of the American College of Cardiology/American Heart Association Task Force on Practice Guidelines. J Am Coll Cardiol 2008;51:172–209.

166. Palmerini T, Marzocchi A, Tamburino C, et al. Temporal pattern of ischemic events in relation to dual antiplatelet therapy in patients with unprotected left main coronary artery stenosis undergoing percutaneous coronary intervention. J Am Coll Cardiol 2009;53:1176-1181.

167. Angiolillo DJ, Fernandez-Ortiz A, Bernardo E et al. Variability in individual responsiveness to clopidogrel: clinical implications, management and future perspectives. J Am Coll Cardiol 2007;49:1505–1516.

168. Angiolillo DJ, Fernandez-Ortiz A, Bernardo E et al. High clopidogrel loading dose during coronary stenting: effects on drug response and interindividual variability. Eur Heart J 2004;25:1903–1910.

169. Cuisset T, Frere C, Quilici J et al. Benefit of a 600-mg loading dose of clopidogrel on platelet reactivity and clinical outcomes in patients with non-ST-segment elevation acute coronary syndrome undergoing coronary stenting. J Am Coll Cardiol 2006;48:1339–1345.

170. Patti G, Colonna G, Pasceri V et al. Randomized trial of high loading dose of clopidogrel for reduction of periprocedural myocardial infarction in patients undergoing coronary intervention: results from the ARMYDA-2 (Antiplatelet therapy for Reduction of Myocardial Damage during Angioplasty) study. Circulation 2005;111:2099–2106.

171. von Beckerath N, Kastrati A, Wieczorek A et al. A double-blind randomized study on platelet aggregation in patients treated with daily dose of 150 or 75 mg of clopidogrel for 30 days. Eur Heart J 2007;28:1814–1819.

172. Angiolillo DJ, Bernardo E, Palazuelos J et al. Functional impact of high clopidogrel maintenance dosing in patients undergoing elective percutaneous coronary interventions. Results of a randomized study. Thromb Haemost 2008;99:161–168.

173. Angiolillo DJ, Shoemaker SB, Desai B et al. Randomized comparison of a high clopidogrel maintenance dose in patients with diabetes mellitus and coronary artery disease: results of the Optimizing Antiplatelet Therapy in Diabetes Mellitus (OPTIMUS) study. Circulation 2007;115:708–716.

174. Angiolillo DJ, Suryadevara S, Capranzano P et al. Antiplatelet drug response variability and the role of the platelet function testing: a pratical guide for interventional cardiologists. Catheter Cardiovasc Interv 2009;73:1–14.

175. Angiolillo DJ. ADP receptor antagonism: what's in the pipeline? Am J Cardiovasc Drugs 2007;7:423–432.

176. Wiviott SD, Braunwald E, Mc Cabe CH et al. Prasugrel versus clopidogrel in patients with acute coronary syndromes. N Engl J Med 2007;357:2001–2015.

177. Palmerini T, Sangiorgi D, Marzocchi A et al. Impact of acute coronary syndromes on two-year clinical outcomes in patients with unprotected left main coronary artery stenosis treated with drug eluting stents: a call for a more powerful antiplatelet therapy? SICI-GISE data

Printed in May 2009